Dance to the Musicals

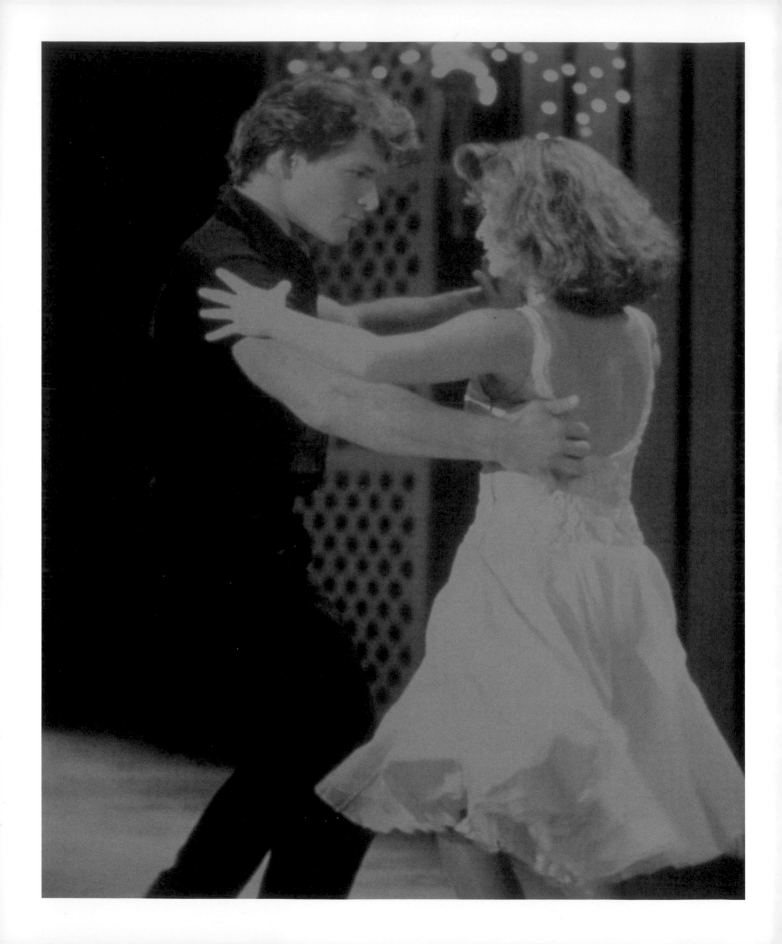

ARLENE PHILLIPS

Dance to the Musicals

K

First published in Great Britain in 2011 by
Kyle Books
23 Howland Street
London, W1T 4AY
www.kylebooks.com

ISBN: 9780857830616

Editor: Judith Hannam
Design: David Rowley
Photography: Gregory King
Dancers: Giorgia Barberi, Hannah Levanne, Callum Powell, Michael de Ritchie and Sue White
Hair and make up: Alana Phillips
Editorial Assistant: Laura Foster
Proofreader: Abi Waters
Production: David Hearn and Nic Jones

A Cataloguing in Publication record for this title is available from the British Library.

Colour reproduction by Altaimage Ltd
Printed and bound in China by Toppan Leefung Printing Ltd

Photographic acknowledgements

page 2: SNAP/Rex Features, page 10: The Moviestore Collection Ltd, pages 22–23: The
Moviestore Collection Ltd, page 32: The Moviestore Collection Ltd, pages 42–43: Everett
Collection/Rex Features, page 50: The Moviestore Collection Ltd, pages 66–67: New Line/
Everett/Rex Features, page 80: Denis O'Regan/CORBIS, page 96: The Moviestore Collection
Ltd, pages 108–109: Paramount/Everett/Rex Features, page 120: The Moviestore Collection
Ltd, page 136: Nils Jorgensen/Rex Features, page 154: The Moviestore Collection Ltd,
pages 168–169: Paramount/Everett/Rex Features, page 178: The Moviestore Collection Ltd,
pages 190–191: The Moviestore Collection Ltd, page 200: The Moviestore Collection Ltd,
pages 212–213: The Moviestore Collection Ltd

contents

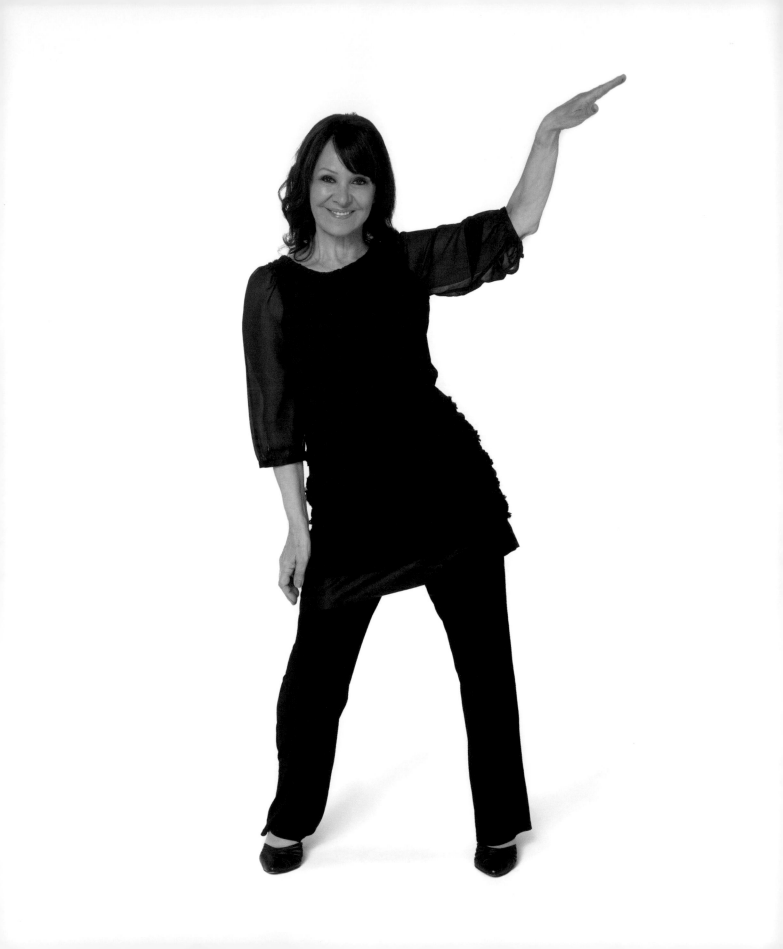

I have to dance to live!

Hi, I'm Arlene Phillips, welcome to my book!

For me, dance is like breathing. It makes me who I am. Although I obviously have no memory of it, I'm told I started dancing as soon as I could walk. Growing up in Manchester, I was lucky to find the best dance teachers and I saw every musical film, ballet and stage show that came to the city. Learning to dance was very hard work because I had to overcome two major obstacles. I didn't have the perfect physique for a dancer. Far from being naturally slender with incredible flexibility, I was stocky and short. I still am. My teachers were very critical. They could have put me off, but their criticism had the opposite effect. It just made me more determined to improve. Dance lessons were expensive. My parents couldn't afford them, so I took any odd jobs I could find to pay the bills. Nothing was going to stop me doing what I loved most in the world. All these years later, I've never stopped dancing, and I've never lost the joy of watching dance – the excitement and tingle when the curtain goes up.

Human beings have danced for centuries. It's a way of communicating without words and a celebration of being alive. Think of maypole dancing, clog dancing, morris dancing, ballroom dancing, line dancing, flamenco, tango, salsa, jive and disco dancing – the list goes on, and demand for classes

'I didn't have the perfect physique for a dancer. Far from being naturally slender with incredible flexibility, I was stocky and short. I still am.'

'Although this is an exercise book, it's about having fun while you get in shape. The routines are all done to musical numbers that everyone will recognise and which lift the spirits.'

grows bigger every year. You don't have to be a professional to feel the joy and freedom dance brings. Watch small children and you'll see them unselfconsciously skipping and dancing. It's the most natural thing in the world. As adults, we've lost that ability to skip and dance. I want to help you find it again. I believe that anyone can dance. Believe me – if you can walk in time to music you can dance.

Although this is an exercise book, it's about having fun while you get in shape. The routines are all danced to musical numbers that everyone will recognise and which lift the spirits. They contain lots of different styles of dance, and although some may look harder than others, they're all broken down into easy-to-follow, step-by-step instructions, so you'll be dancing along in no time! They are a great workout, either to do on your own, in which case you can focus on your improvement each week, or to do with friends, so you can encourage each other and feel like you are at your very own dance class.

Being fit isn't just about having a healthy heart and strong muscles, it's also about connecting your brain to quickly send messages to your arms and legs, so that your mind remains young and active along with your body.

Accompanying the book, you'll find a free DVD of four of the routines, featuring step-by-step instructions followed by the routines danced to the music. Remember they're fast, but you'll be joining in with the professionals sooner than you think.

Before you begin

Start by making sure you're wearing comfortable clothes that are easy to move in, and suitable footwear such as trainers or low-heeled shoes that aren't going to slip off. You'll need to dance on a non-slip surface, and remember to move all the furniture out of the way to give yourself plenty of room.

You'll need to learn routines 1 and 10 first, as these are the warm-up and the cool-down. It's important you do these at the beginning and end of every session. Learning the steps one by one, then putting them together will make the routines easier to follow and they'll become second nature in no time, plus all the routines have simple counts to help you keep in time with the music. Once you have learnt the routine thoroughly, you can repeat it again from the beginning, as this will help you increase your stamina. Start with five minutes each day and build up.

So are you ready? Let's get those dancing shoes on!

Arlene Phillips

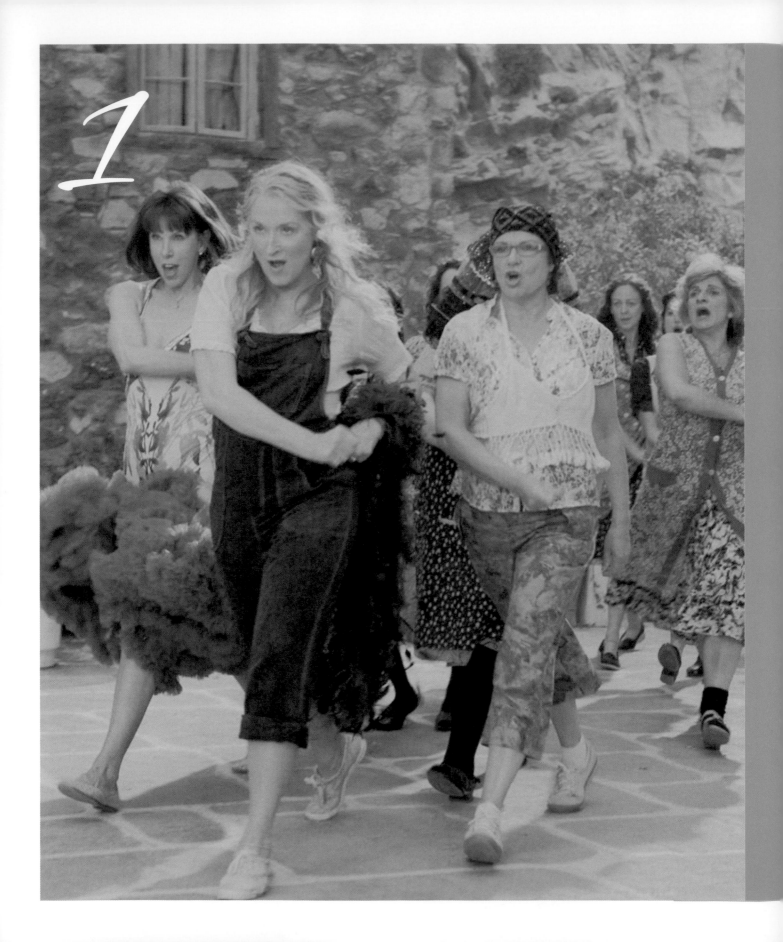

Mamma Mia

Mamma Mia

Written by Benny Andersson and Björn Ulvaeus

It's about having a good time. It's a dance routine which will set you aglow. Keep at it, you won't even have to think about which step comes next

Mamma Mia was choreographed by a good friend and colleague of mine, Anthony van Laast, who I collaborated with on a BBC 1 Saturday night entertainment called *The Hot Shoe Show*. I don't know anybody who doesn't love *Mamma Mia*, but in the days before the first night I remember Anthony describing to me that awful feeling you get when you think a show isn't going to work. Not for one moment did he think he had a hit on his hands, or a production that would eventually go all over the world – Europe, North America, South America, China, Japan and Korea. Nor could anyone in their wildest dreams have imagined that it would be turned into a smash–hit film starring Meryl Streep.

There's not that much dancing in the show, but the music cries out to be danced to. It's an integral part of the great 80s disco era. I doubt any other group apart from Abba has spawned so many tribute bands. Their life–enhancing music is known worldwide, just like Andrew Lloyd Webber's *Cats* and *Phantom of the Opera*, and if you visit a hotel lounge anywhere in the world, however isolated, you're likely to hear one of their songs being played.

The rhythm in 'Mamma Mia' is so clear, which makes it easy to dance to for anyone who has trouble keeping in time with the beat! Finding a natural rhythm is often the most difficult thing for a non–dancer. But if Meryl Streep and Julie Walters can dance in time to the music and connect one step to another then you can too! This routine is perfect for a warm up session. It's about having a good time. It's a dance routine which will set you aglow. Keep at it, and you won't even have to think about which step comes next. It will exercise your whole body and your brain will say a big thank you too!

This is a good cardiovascular routine, working all the major muscle groups. A great workout to practise on a daily basis as this will give you great stamina, good coordination skills and a fitness level that will help you maintain a healthy quality of life. 'Mamma Mia' a day keeps the doctor away!

Starting position: right leg forward, with your hands in boxing fists

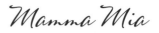

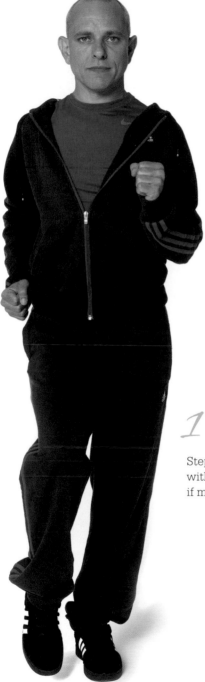

1

Step onto your right foot, with your hands in fists, as if marching, count 1

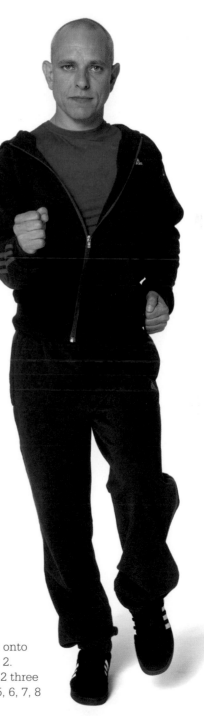

2

Still marching, step onto your left foot, count 2. Repeat steps 1 and 2 three times, counts 3, 4, 5, 6, 7, 8

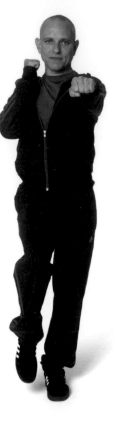

3

Continue marching on the spot, punch forward with your right arm, left arm bent with your hand in a fist facing in, count 1

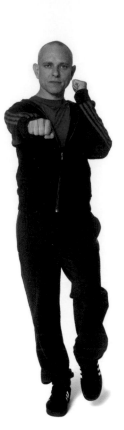

4

Continue marching on the spot, punch forward with your left arm, right arm bent with your hand in a fist facing in, count 2. Repeat steps 3 and 4 three times, counts 3, 4, 5, 6, 7, 8. Repeat steps 1–4

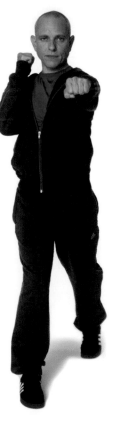

5

Spring your left foot forward, keeping your right foot back, and punch forward with your right arm, count 1

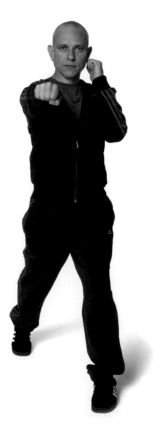

6

Spring to change feet, punch forward with your left arm, pulling your right arm back into your body, your hand in a fist facing in, count 2.
Repeat steps 5 and 6 three times, counts 3, 4, 5, 6, 7, 8

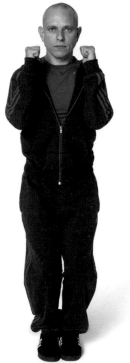

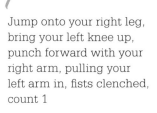

7

Jump onto your right leg, bring your left knee up, punch forward with your right arm, pulling your left arm in, fists clenched, count 1

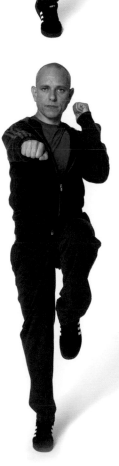

8

Jump, bringing your feet together, bend your knees, both arms bent with your fists clenched beside your cheeks, count 2

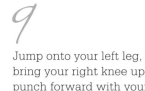

9

Jump onto your left leg, bring your right knee up, punch forward with your left arm, right arm in, count 3

10

Jump bringing your feet together, count 4. Repeat steps 7–10, counts 5, 6, 7, 8. Repeat steps 5–10

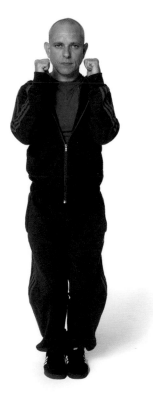

Imagine you have a
skipping rope, jump in the
air with your feet together,
making small circles with
your arms, keeping your
elbows tucked into your
sides, count 'and'

Land with your feet together,
knees bent, and continue to
make circles with your arms,
bringing them lower, count 1.
Repeat steps 11 and 12
seven times, counts and 2,
and 3, and 4, and 5, and 6,
and 7, and 8

13

Continue circling your arms, land onto your right foot, count 1

14

Land on your left foot, count 2. Repeat steps 13 and 14 three times, counts 3, 4, 5, 6, 7, 8. Repeat steps 11–14

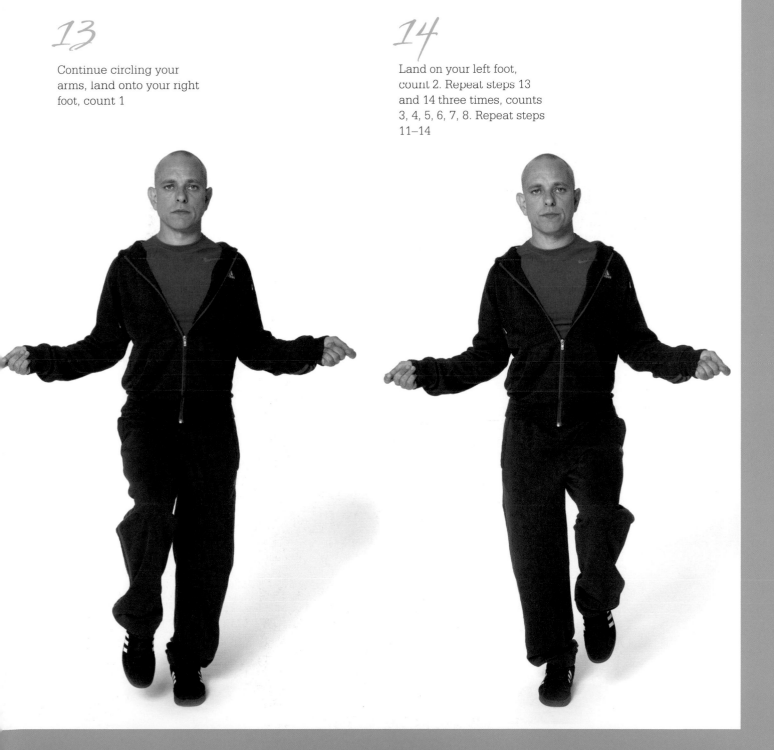

15

Slide your weight onto
your right leg, leaving your
left leg out to the side,
keeping your arms bent,
and your fists close to your
cheeks, count 1

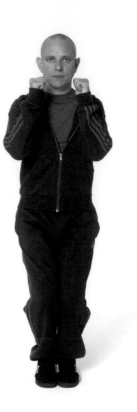

16

Bring your left leg to join
the right, keeping your
arms in the same position,
count 2

17

Slide your weight onto
your left leg, leaving your
right leg out to the side,
keeping your arms bent,
and your fists close to your
cheeks, count 3

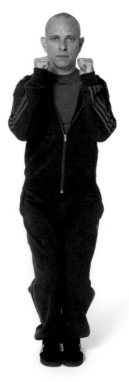

18

Bring your right leg to join
your left, keeping your
arms in the same position,
count 4. Repeat steps
15–18, counts 5, 6, 7, 8

19

Slide your weight onto your right leg, leaving your left leg out to the side, keeping your arms bent, and your fists close to your cheeks, count 1

20

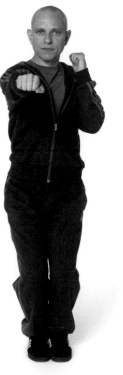

Bring your left leg to join the right, and punch forward with your left arm, count 2

21

Slide your weight onto your left leg, bringing your left arm in, count 3

22

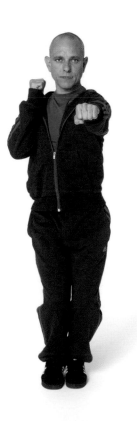

Bring your right leg to join your left, and punch forward with your right arm, count 4. Repeat steps 19–22, counts 5, 6, 7, 8. Repeat steps 15–22

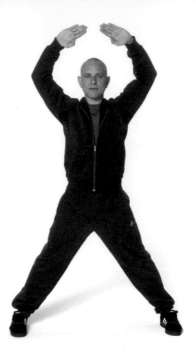

23

Jump, with your feet apart, letting your arms go out and up to the side, finishing with your hands above your head, count 1

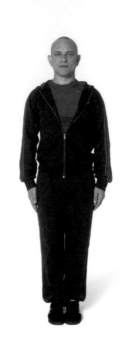

24

Jump, bringing your feet back together, your arms down by your sides, count 2

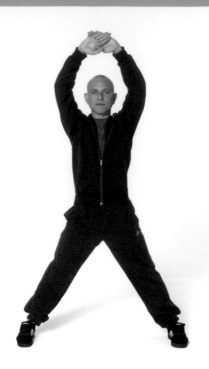

25

Jump with your feet apart, lifting your arms up in front of your body, and finishing with them above your head, hands together, count 3

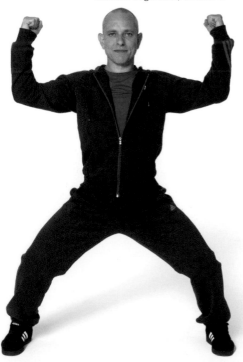

26

Jump bringing your feet back together, arms down, count 4. Repeat steps 23–26, counts 5, 6, 7, 8

27

Jump feet apart, knees bent, your arms raised strongly to the side, count 1

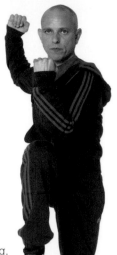

28

Jump onto your right leg, lift your left leg to the front, and take your right elbow to your left knee, count 2

29

Jump feet apart, your arms raised strongly to the side, count 3

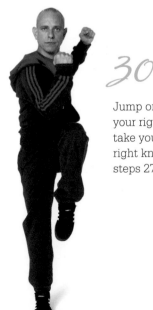

30

Jump onto your left leg, lift your right leg forward, and take your left elbow to your right knee, count 4. Repeat steps 27 and 28, counts 5, 6

31

Step forward onto your left leg, raising both arms up, count 7

32

Bring the right foot next to the left, both fists on hips, count 8.
Repeat steps 23–32

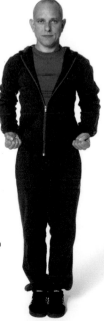

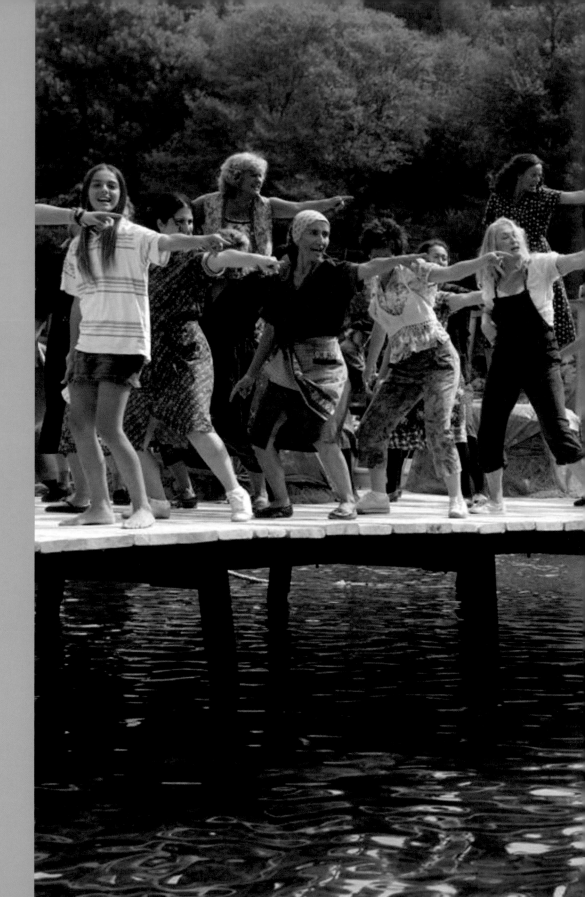

This image from *Mamma Mia* proves that you're never too young or too old to join in and dance!

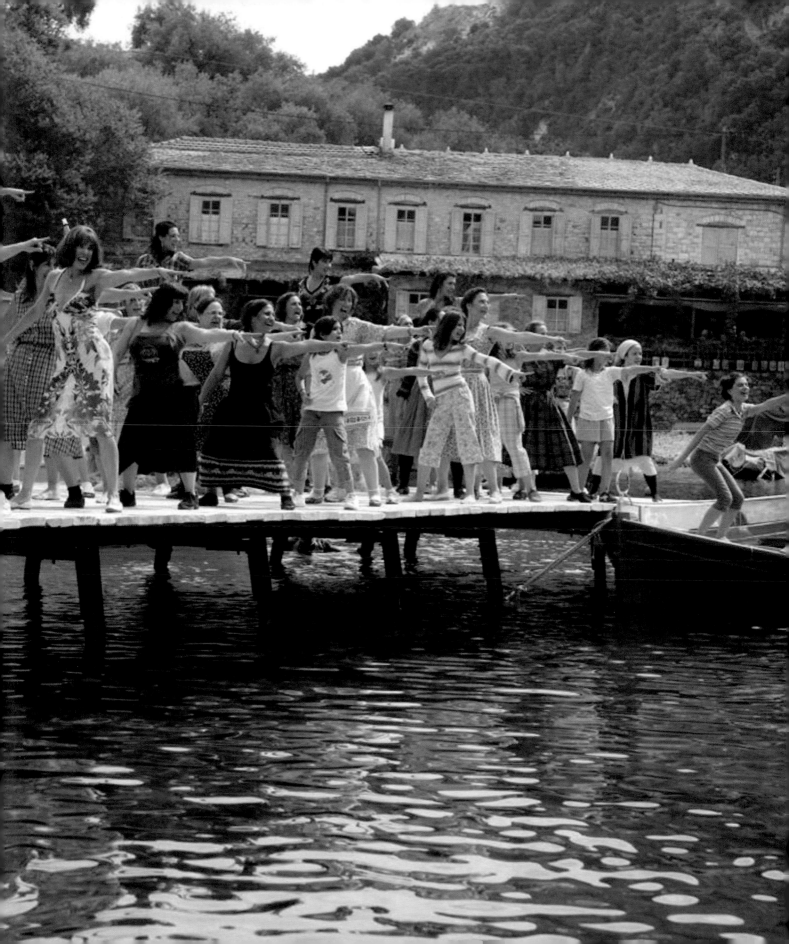

33

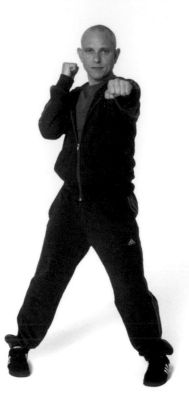

Step onto your right foot, and punch forward with your right arm, count 1

34

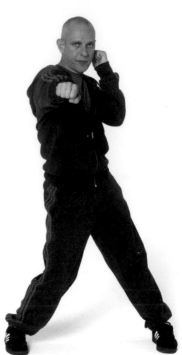

Step onto your left foot, and punch forward with your left arm, count 2. Repeat steps 33 and 34, counts 3, 4

35

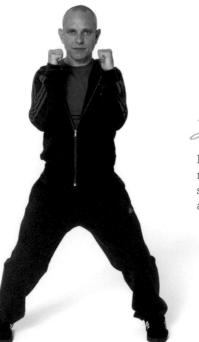

Bend both legs, keeping both arms in, and fists by your cheeks, count 5

36

Put your weight onto your right leg, right arm to the side, and keep your left arm in place, count 'and'

37

Come up onto a straight right leg, tap your left foot, and make a hook punch with your right arm, count 6

38

Bend both knees, keeping both arms in, count 7

39

Put your weight onto your left leg, take your left arm to the side, keeping your right arm in place, count 'and'

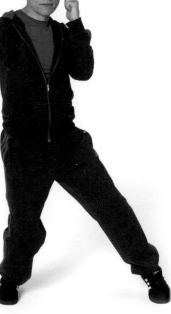

40

Come up onto a straight left leg, tap your right foot, and make a hook punch with your left arm, count 8. Repeat steps 33–40, counts 1, 2, 3, 4, 5, 'and', 6, 7, 'and', 8

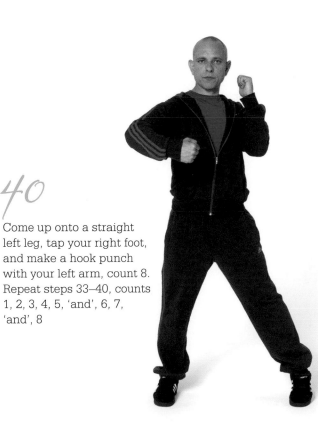

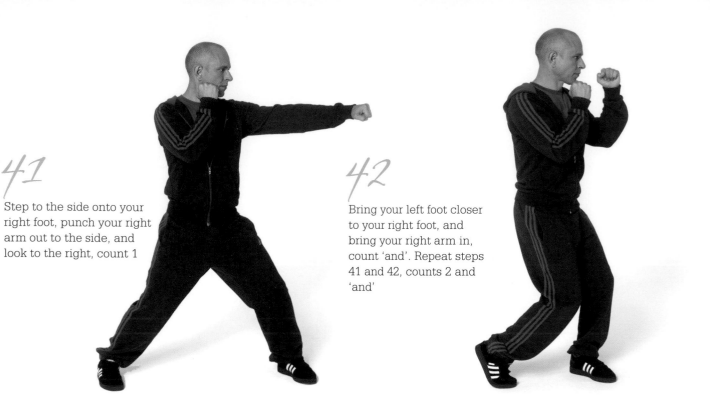

41
Step to the side onto your right foot, punch your right arm out to the side, and look to the right, count 1

42
Bring your left foot closer to your right foot, and bring your right arm in, count 'and'. Repeat steps 41 and 42, counts 2 and 'and'

43
Step onto your right leg, and punch your right arm out to the side, count 3

44
Punch forward with your left arm, bring your right arm back, and stretch your legs, count 4

45

Step back onto your left foot, bend your knees, and bring both arms in, count 5

46

Step in with your right foot, and come up to straight legs, count 6

47

Step onto your left foot, and bend both your knees, count 7

48

Turn your body to the front, and straighten both your legs, count 8

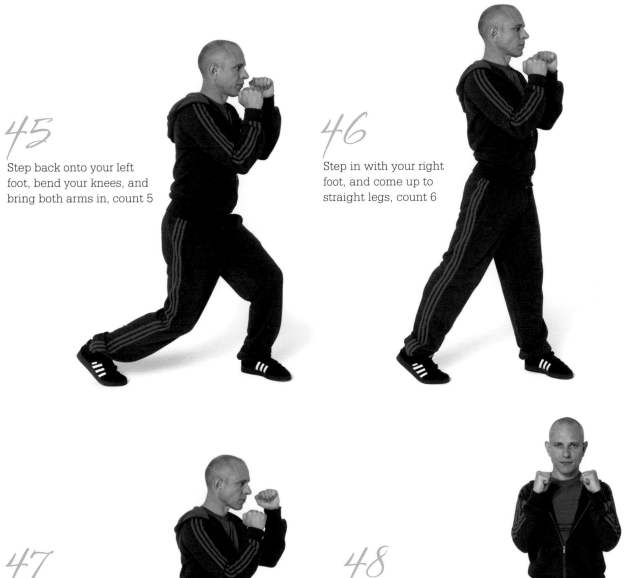

49

Step to the side onto your left foot, punch your left arm out to the side, and look to the left, count 1

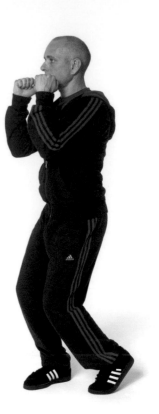

50

Bring your right foot closer to your left foot, and bring your left arm in, count 'and'. Repeat steps 49 and 50, counts 2 'and'

51

Step onto your left leg, and punch your left arm out to the side, count 3

52

Punch your right arm forward, bring your left arm into your body, and stretch your legs, count 4

53

Step back onto your right foot, bend your knees, both arms in, count 5

54

Step in with your left foot, come up to straight legs, count 6

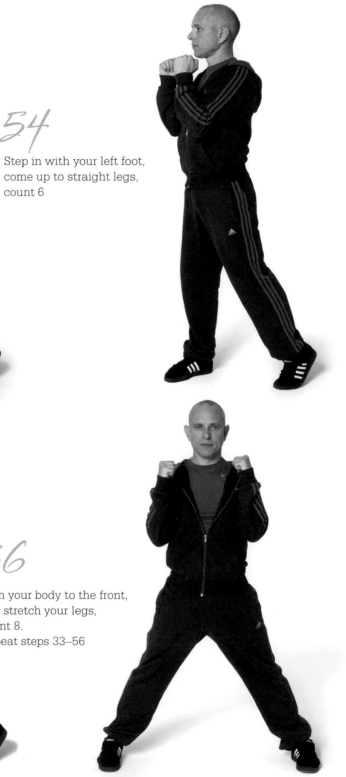

55

Step onto your left foot, and bend both your knees, count 7

56

Turn your body to the front, and stretch your legs, count 8.
Repeat steps 33–56

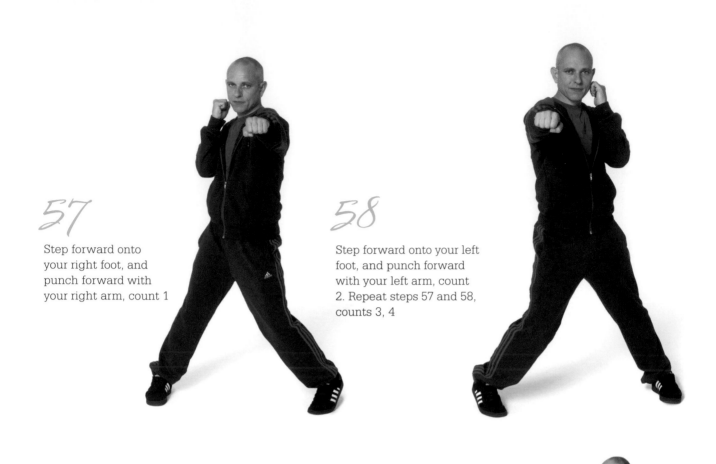

57

Step forward onto your right foot, and punch forward with your right arm, count 1

58

Step forward onto your left foot, and punch forward with your left arm, count 2. Repeat steps 57 and 58, counts 3, 4

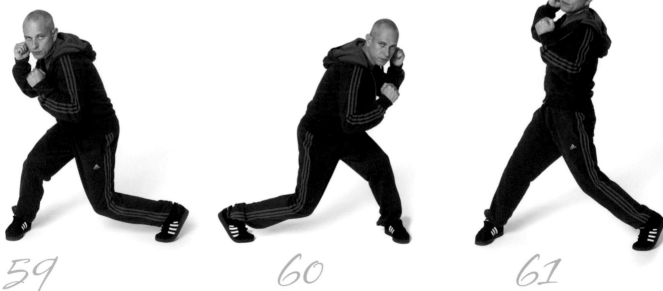

59

Bend both your knees, and drop your right shoulder down to your left knee, count 5

60

Bring your left shoulder down to your right knee, both knees bent, count 6

61

Punch upwards with your right arm, making a fist, switching legs at the same time, count 7

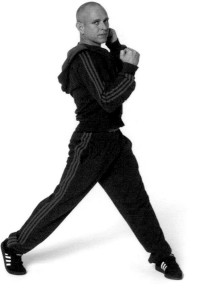

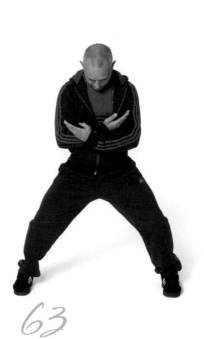

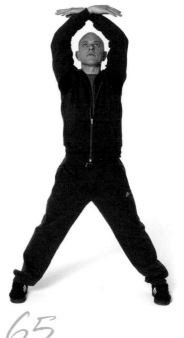

 62

Switch to the other side, punching upwards with your left arm, making a fist, count 8. Repeat steps 57–62

63

Deep breath in, feet apart, arms crossed in front of chest, palms facing upwards count 1 . . .

65

. . . and up, counts 5, 6, 7 and 8

 64

Continue moving your arms upwards to finish above your head, counts 1, 2, 3 and 4

66

Slowly breathe out, and take your arms back down, counts 1, 2, 3 and 4. Finish with your arms by your sides in a relaxed position, counts 5, 6, 7 , 8

As you build your stamina, repeat the entire routine from the beginning

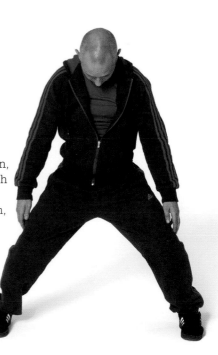

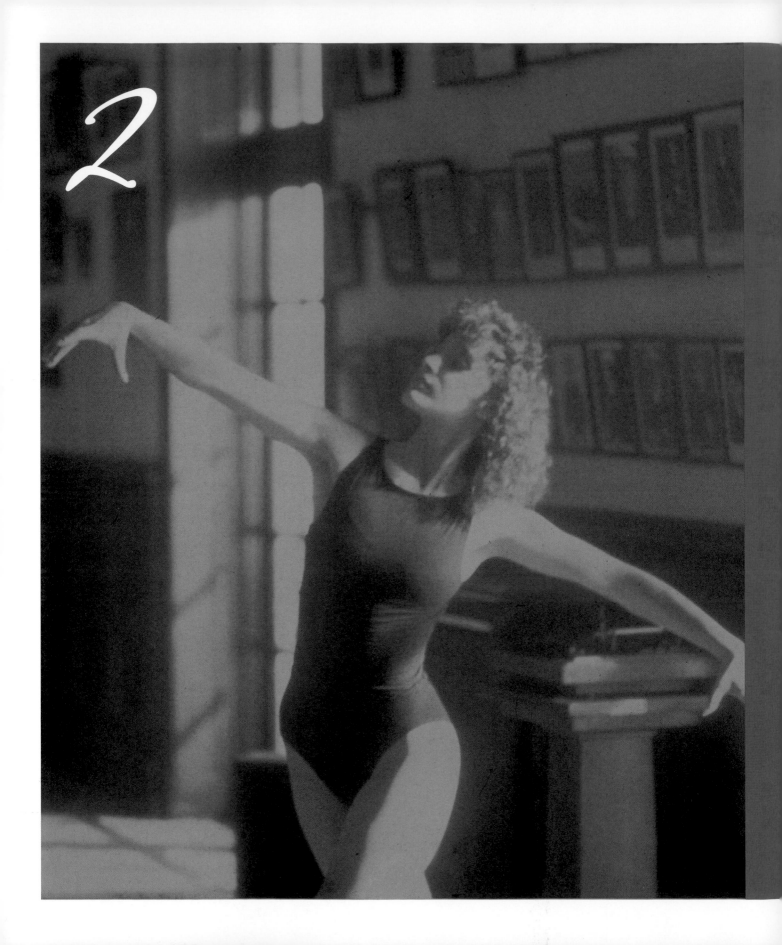

Flashdance

What a Feeling

Written by Giorgio Moroder, Keith Forsey and Irene Cara

'What A Feeling' says everything there is to say about dance. It's a combination of basic exercise with a jazz feel, leading to some familiar 80s dance moves

When I was in America in 1983, choreographing the film Annie, I got a call to meet the producer Tom Hedley, who was about to make the film Flashdance. After several meetings, it was finally down to two choreographers. I didn't get the job, and I thought no more of it, but several years later, Tom called again to ask me to choreograph the stage musical. The story focuses on Alex Owens, an 18-year-old girl who by day works in the steel works and by night moonlights as a dancer at Mawby's Bar and dreams of studying at the prestigious Pittsburgh Dance and Repertory Company   a girl after my own heart! I loved the movie, but, as a choreographer, I knew my hardest challenge would be the finale, which, in the film, had five different dance doubles. Where would I find one girl who could do it all? We auditioned and kept coming back to Victoria Hamilton Barrett. Although she had done many West End shows as the lead and was a fantastic actress and a great singer, she wasn't first and foremost a dancer. What I wanted was a phenomenal dancer, but every really talented dancer who auditioned couldn't act the part. The girl playing Alex has to be a good strong storyteller as, without that, the end routine doesn't pay off. Victoria eventually proved herself to be the outstanding candidate. That final routine was so tough, but one she managed to pull off, and the audiences loved her. 'What A Feeling' says everything there is to say about dance. My routine is a basic exercise with a jazz feel, with familiar 80s dance moves that will tone your waistline.

The first part of this routine will improve your torso strength while the second part will test bums, tums and arms with its energetic dance moves. What a Feeling!

Starting position: stand straight with your left foot touching your right, arms to the side and prepare to open your left foot to the side

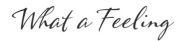

Part 1

1

Stretch your right arm over your head with a double bounce, counts 1, 2

2

Stretch your left arm over your head with a double bounce, counts 3, 4

3

Reach out with your right arm, bending at the waist, but keeping your back straight, with a double bounce, counts 5, 6

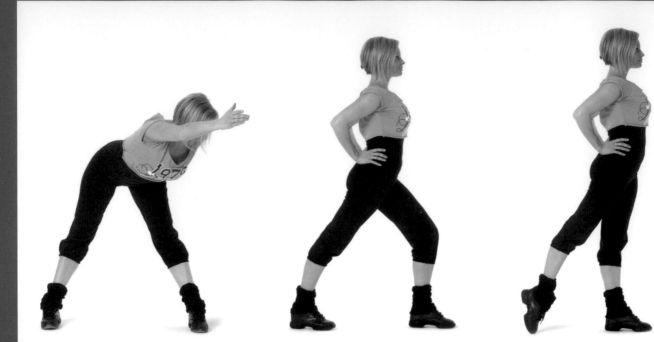

4

Reach out with your left arm, keeping your back straight, with a double bounce, counts 7, 8. Repeat steps 1–4

5

Turn to the right, stretch your left leg, keeping your heel on the floor, count 1

6

Lift your left heel off the floor, point your toes and stretch both legs, count 2. Repeat steps 5 and 6, counts 3, 4

7

Push your left heel into the floor, and raise both arms, counts 5, hold 6

8

Turn to face the front, opening your arms to the side, counts 7, hold 8

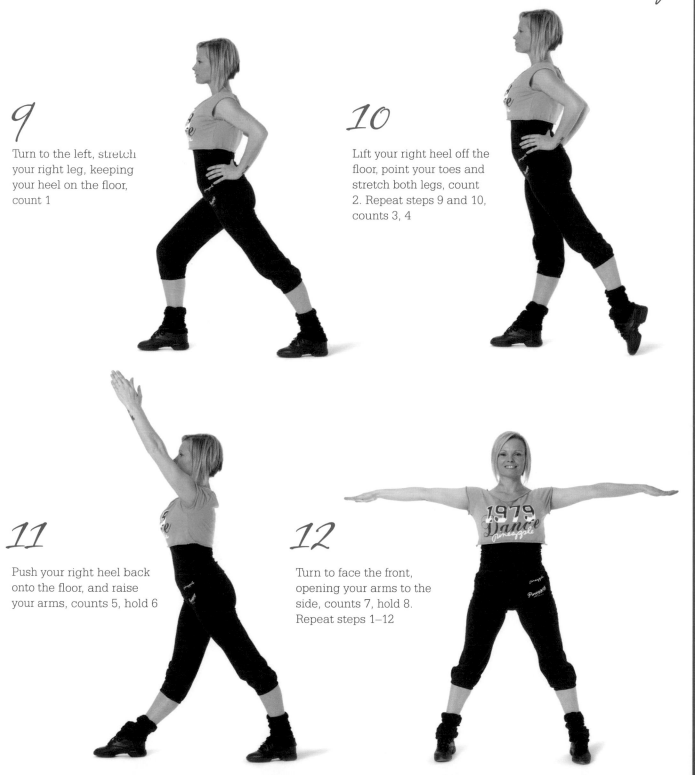

9

Turn to the left, stretch your right leg, keeping your heel on the floor, count 1

10

Lift your right heel off the floor, point your toes and stretch both legs, count 2. Repeat steps 9 and 10, counts 3, 4

11

Push your right heel back onto the floor, and raise your arms, counts 5, hold 6

12

Turn to face the front, opening your arms to the side, counts 7, hold 8. Repeat steps 1–12

Part 2

13

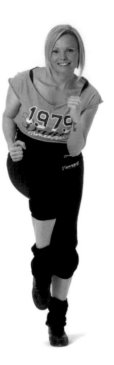

Run, putting your weight onto your right leg, count 1

14

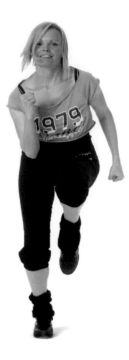

Then onto your left leg, count 2. Repeat steps 13 and 14, counts 3, 4

15

Step out to the side onto your right leg, bringing your left arm across your body, count 5

16

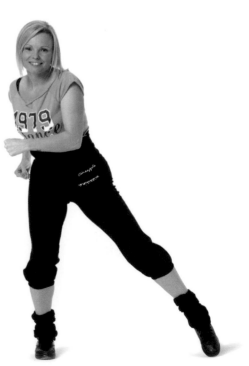

Step out to the side onto your left leg, bringing your right arm across your body, count 6. Repeat steps 15 and 16, counts 7, 8

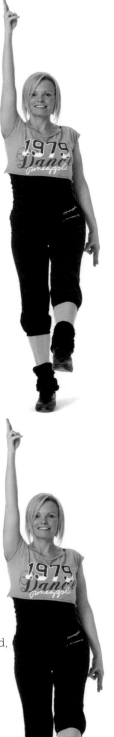

17

Kick your right leg forward, and raise your left arm, count 1

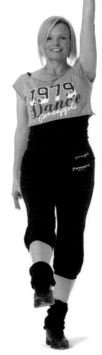

18

Kick your left leg forward, and raise your right arm, count 2

19

Kick your right leg forward, and raise your left arm, count 3

20

Bring your right leg in, count 'and'

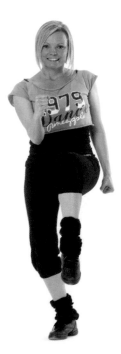

21

Kick your right leg forward, and raise your left arm, count 4

22

Kick your left leg forward, and raise your right arm, count 5

23

Kick your right leg forward, and raise your left arm, count 6

24

Kick your left leg forward, and raise your right arm, count 7

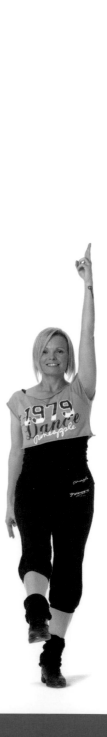

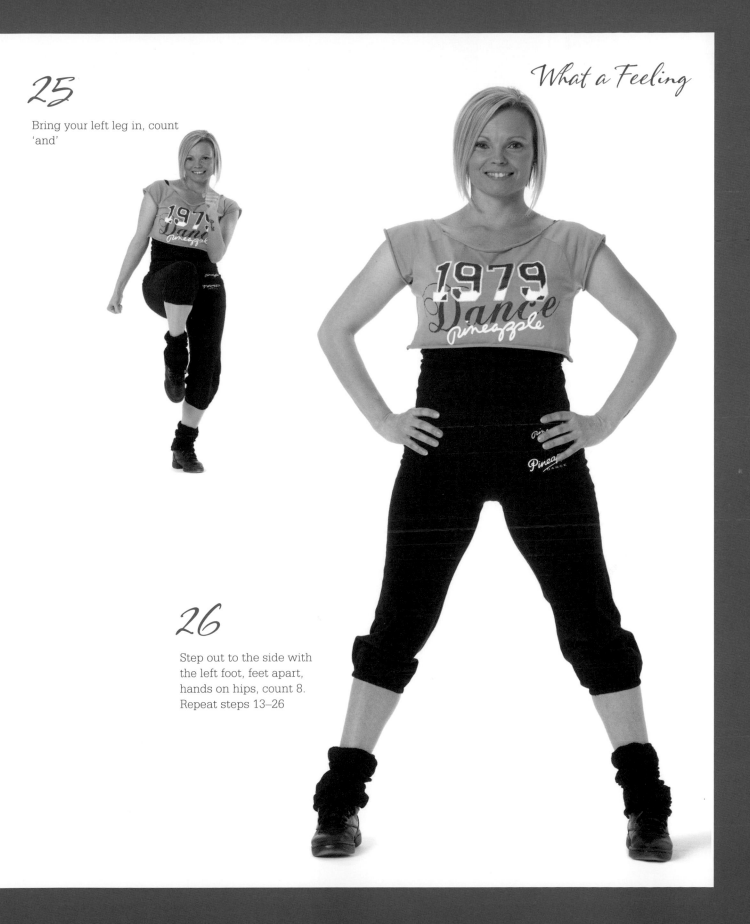

25

Bring your left leg in, count
'and'

26

Step out to the side with
the left foot, feet apart,
hands on hips, count 8.
Repeat steps 13–26

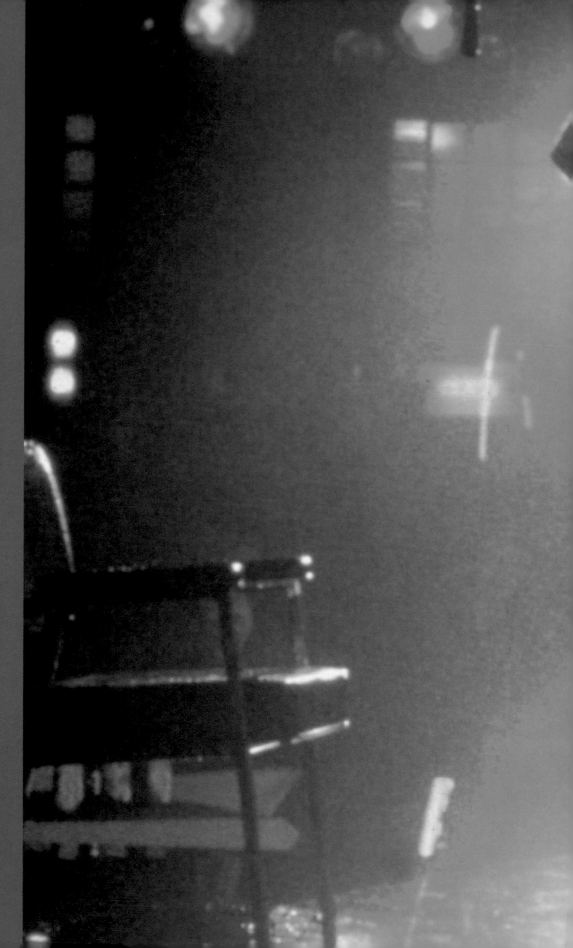

An iconic moment from the film, just before Alex reaches the climax of the dance, when she sits in the chair and releases the water from above

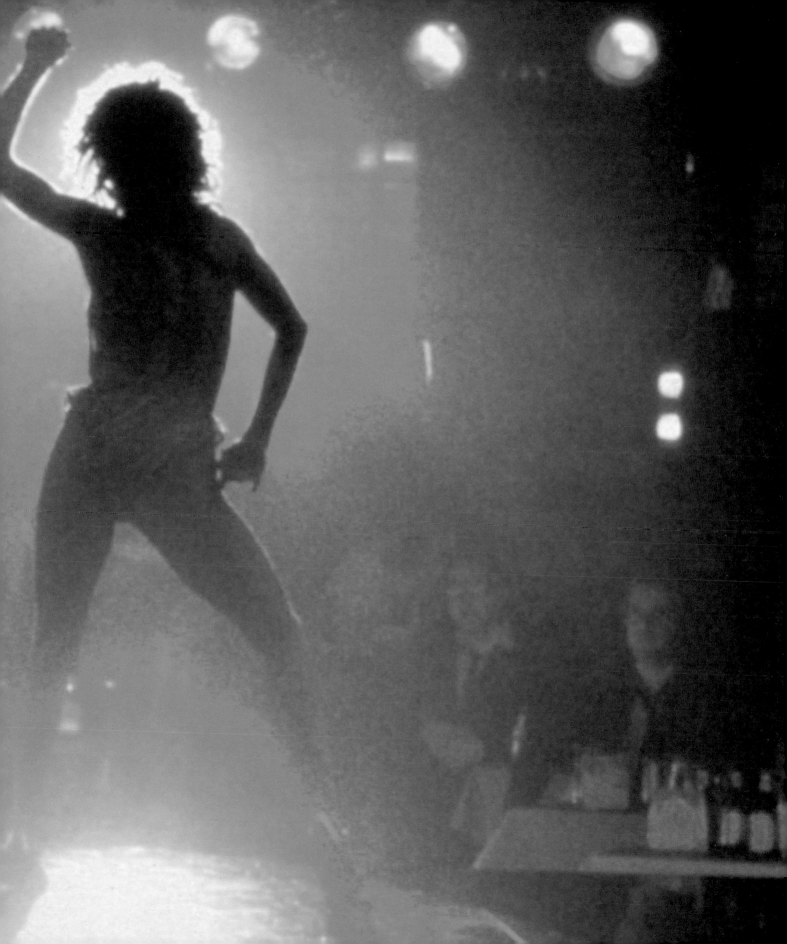

Part 3

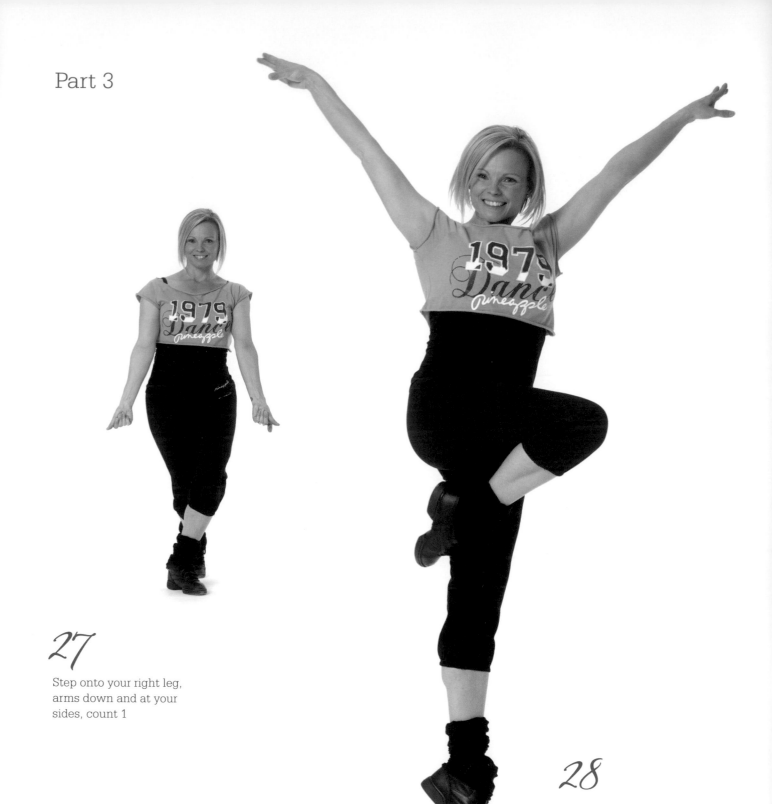

27

Step onto your right leg, arms down and at your sides, count 1

28

Jump on your right foot, bring your left knee up and raise your arms to the side, count 2

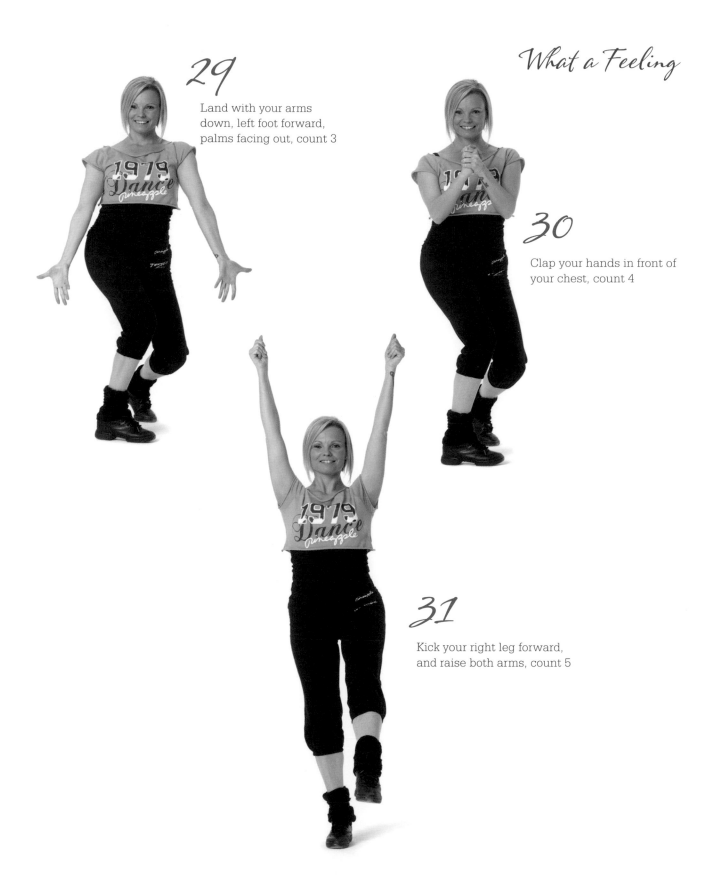

29

Land with your arms down, left foot forward, palms facing out, count 3

30

Clap your hands in front of your chest, count 4

31

Kick your right leg forward, and raise both arms, count 5

Part 4

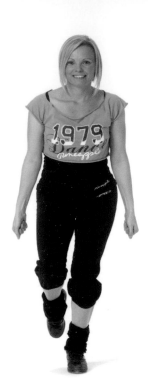

32

Jump on to your right leg, bring your arms down to the side, count 'and'

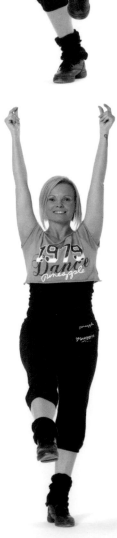

33

Step back onto your left leg, and raise your right knee, count 6

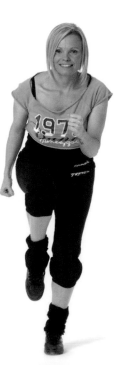

34

Step forward onto your right leg and raise your left knee, count 'and'

35

Kick your left leg forward and raise both arms, count 7

36

Drop onto to your left leg,
and bring both arms down,
count 'and'

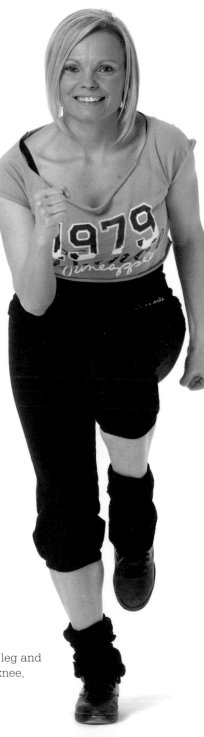

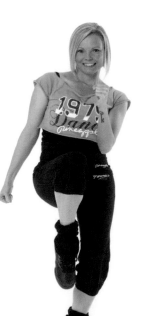

37

Step back onto your right
leg and raise your left
knee, count 8

38

Drop to your left leg and
raise your right knee,
count 'and'

Part 4

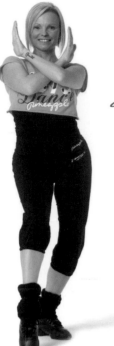

39

Step back onto your right leg, crossing your arms underneath your face, count 1

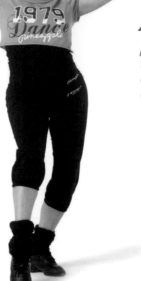

40

Slide your hands, palms down, beside your face, count 2

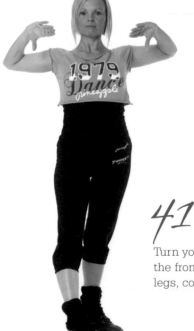

41

Turn your palms to face the front, and stretch both legs, count 3

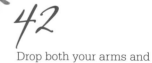

42

Drop both your arms and your head forward, count 4

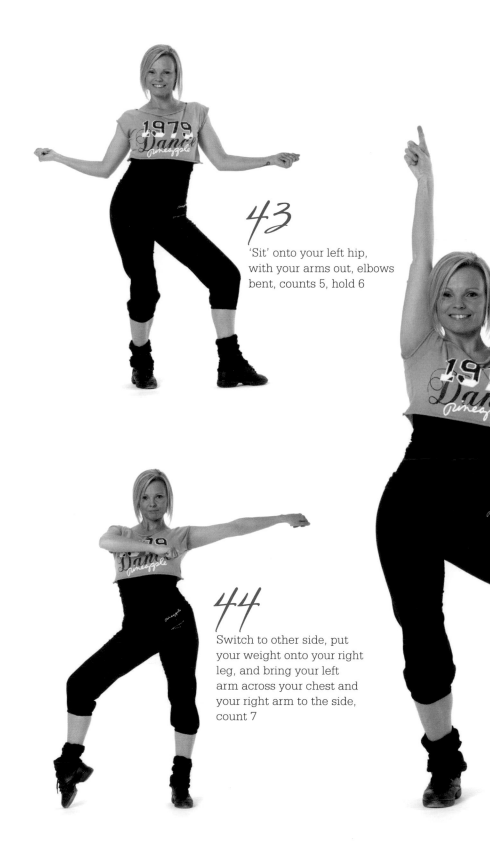

43
'Sit' onto your left hip, with your arms out, elbows bent, counts 5, hold 6

44
Switch to other side, put your weight onto your right leg, and bring your left arm across your chest and your right arm to the side, count 7

45
Bring your weight back onto your left leg, raise your left arm up, and put your right arm behind your head, count 8

As you build your stamina, repeat the entire routine from the beginning

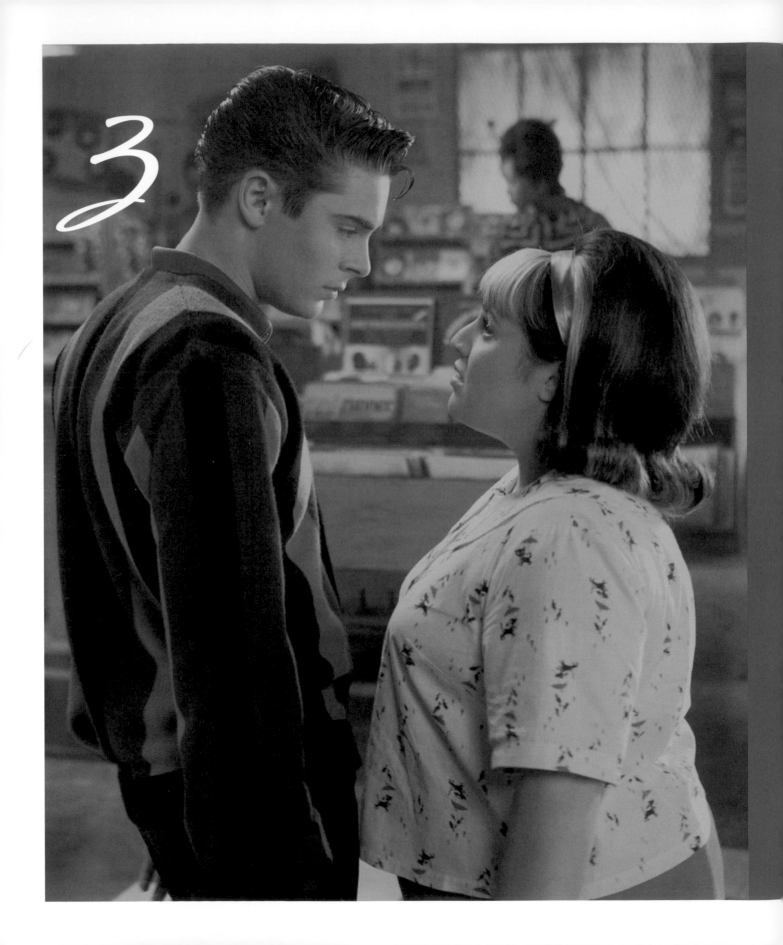

Hairspray

You Can't Stop the Beat

Written by Marc Shaiman and Scott Wittman

I've always been a huge fan of John Waters and, by chance, I was in New York for meetings when the show opened on Broadway. Obviously I hot-footed it to the theatre as soon as I could. I was wearing my most comfortable walking shoes and casual clothes, but sitting in the theatre I was surrounded by a front stalls audience weighed down by diamonds and glitz. I realised immediately it was the hottest ticket in town and had 'hit' written all over it. Anyone who was anyone had come to see *Hairspray*. All around me they were laughing, shouting and having a ball. But all I kept thinking was how over the top it was. For me, the show felt garish. I fell in love with the performances and the music, but it still felt a bit like the Emperor's New Clothes. I couldn't quite bring myself to get involved in the hysteria. What had this diamond-clad audience seen that I hadn't?

When *Hairspray* opened in London, Michael Ball starred as Edna Turnblad. He's someone to whom I'm very close, both as a friend and a choreographer, and this time, with his star performance, I loved it. Everything I'd felt was not quite right in New York worked in London, where it was played more for real – not just for laughs. It had a truth to it. So I kept on going back. This was one jumping, screaming, joyful production that touched me in a way that the Broadway show hadn't.

It's impossible to keep still to the up-tempo music of 'You Can't Stop the Beat'. You'll want to clap, jump, dance and skip. It will lift your mood. So as it says in the lyrics, 'Get on your feet and join the party.' This is a wake-up, shake-up routine to get your heart pumping!

It's impossible to keep still to the up-tempo music of 'You Can't Stop the Beat'. This is a wake-up, shake-up routine to get your heart pumping!

This is a challenging dance routine that involves a good level of coordination. It will help build muscular strength in your legs and bottom. Feel the heat as you get the beat! Rock on!

Starting position: feet together, lift arms and open hands

1

Jump to the side onto your right foot, bending your left knee and crossing your arms low down, left over right, count 1

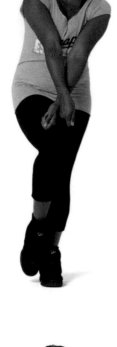

2

Transfer your weight onto the ball of your left foot, and lift your right foot off the floor, count 'and'

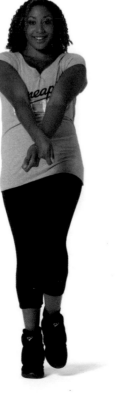

3

Bounce your weight back onto your right foot, and lift your left foot off the floor, count 2

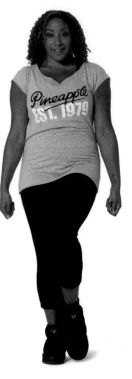

4

Jump onto your left foot, and bring both arms down by your sides, count 3

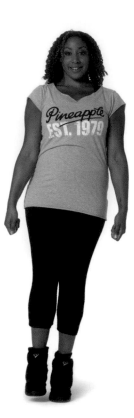

5

Transfer your weight onto the ball of your right foot, count 'and'

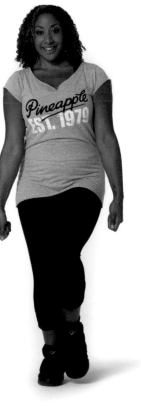

6

Bounce your weight back onto your left foot, and lift your right foot off the floor, count 4.
Repeat steps 1–6, counts 5, 'and', 6, 7, 'and', 8

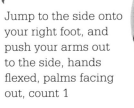

7

Jump to the side onto your right foot, and push your arms out to the side, hands flexed, palms facing out, count 1

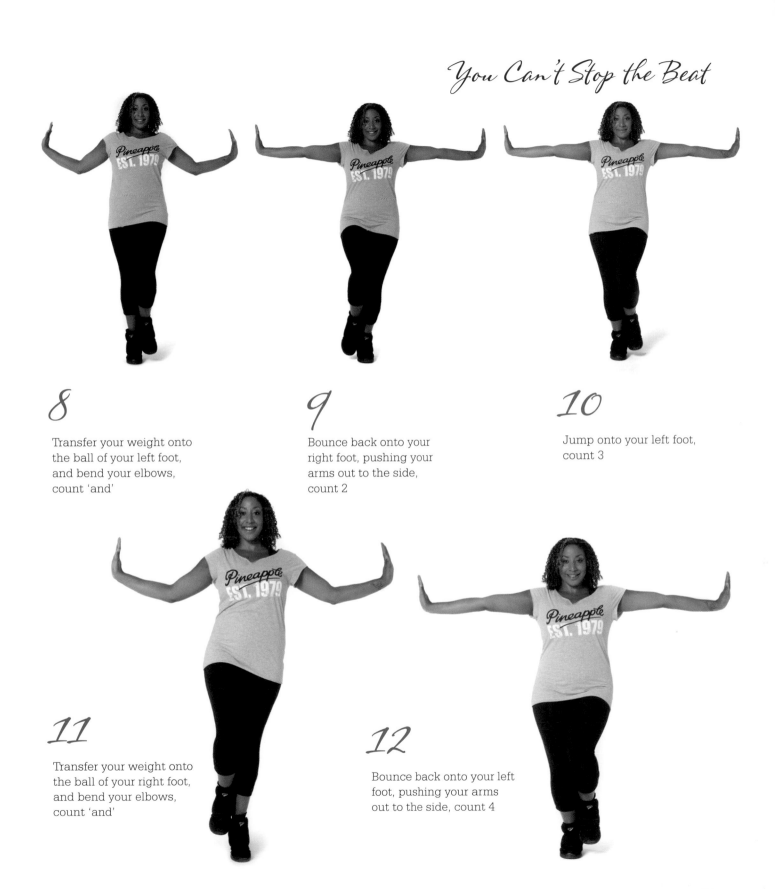

8

Transfer your weight onto the ball of your left foot, and bend your elbows, count 'and'

9

Bounce back onto your right foot, pushing your arms out to the side, count 2

10

Jump onto your left foot, count 3

11

Transfer your weight onto the ball of your right foot, and bend your elbows, count 'and'

12

Bounce back onto your left foot, pushing your arms out to the side, count 4

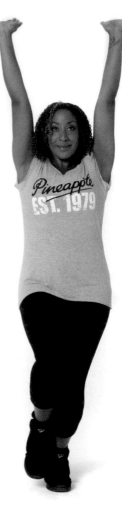

13

Jump onto your right foot, pushing your arms straight up with flexed hands, count 5

14

Transfer your weight onto the ball of your left foot, and bend your elbows, count 'and'

15

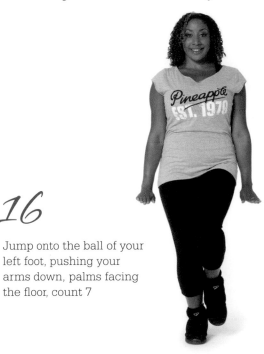

Bounce back onto your right foot, pushing your arms straight up with flexed hands, count 6

16

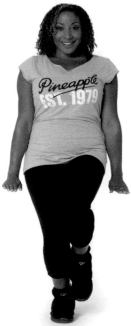

Jump onto the ball of your left foot, pushing your arms down, palms facing the floor, count 7

17

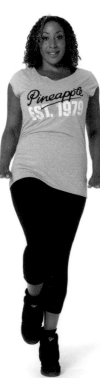

Transfer your weight onto the ball of your right foot, and bend your elbows, count 'and'

18

Bounce back onto your left foot, pushing your arms down, count 8.
Repeat steps 1–18

19

Step forward with your right foot, putting your weight onto your front leg, and bend your elbows, raising your left arm and lowering your right, your hands in fists, count 1

20

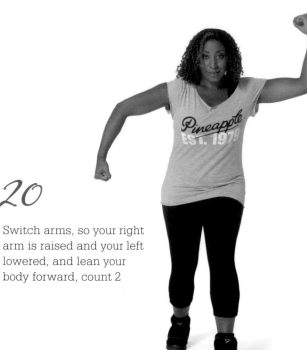

Switch arms, so your right arm is raised and your left lowered, and lean your body forward, count 2

21

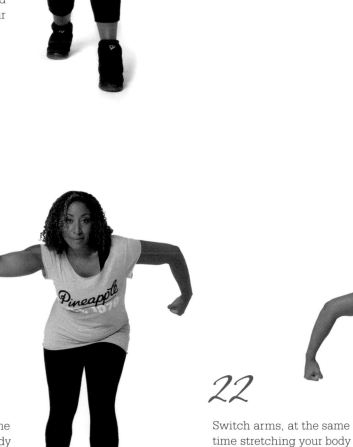

Switch arms, at the same time stretching your body further forward, count 3

22

Switch arms, at the same time stretching your body all the way forward, count 4

Transfer your weight onto
your back leg, bringing
your body upright,
switching arms so that
your left arm is raised
and your right is lowered,
count 5

24

Switch arms, so that
your right arm is raised
and your left is lowered,
leaning backwards,
count 6

25

Switch arms, so that your
left arm is raised and your
right is lowered, bringing
your body upright, count 7

26

Switch arms, so that
your right arm is raised
and your left is lowered,
leaning backwards,
count 8

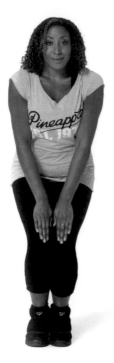

27

Bring your right foot in to join the left, bend your knees, and place both hands, palms flat, on your thighs, count 1

28

Twist your body to the left and, leaning forwards, push your arms out to the corner with flexed hands, both legs straight, count 2

29

Twist back to face the front, bend your knees, and place your hands, palms flat, on your thighs, count 3

31

Twist back to face the front, bend your knees, and place your hands, palms flat, on your thighs, count 7

30

Twist your body to the right and, leaning forwards, push your arms out to the corner with flexed hands, both legs straight, count 4.
Repeat steps 27 and 28, counts 5, 6

32

Push your arms straight up with flexed hands, both knees straight, count 8

33

Step forward with your
left foot, putting your
weight onto your front leg,
and bend your elbows,
raising your right arm and
lowering your left, your
hands in fists, count 1

34

Switch arms, so your left
arm is raised and your
right lowered, and lean
your body forward,
count 2

35

Switch arms, at the same
time stretching your body
further forward, count 3

36

Switch arms again, and stretch your body all the way forward, count 4

37

Bring your body upright, and switch arms so the right is raised and the left is lowered, count 5

38

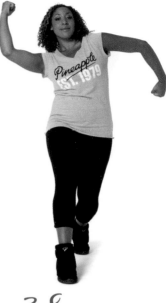

Switch arms, so the left is raised and the right is lowered, and lean backwards, count 6

39

Switch arms, so that your right arm is raised and your left is lowered, and bring your body upright, count 7

40

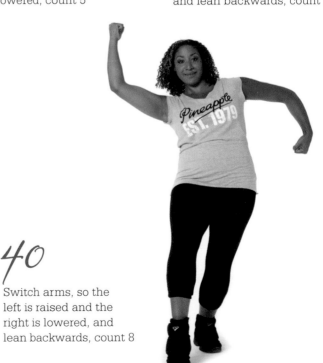

Switch arms, so the left is raised and the right is lowered, and lean backwards, count 8

41

Bring your left foot in to join the right, bend your knees, both hands on your thighs, palms flat, count 1

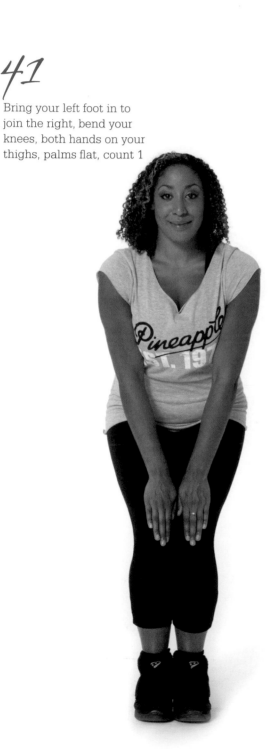

42

Twist your body to the right and, leaning forwards, push your arms out to the corner with flexed hands, both legs straight, count 2

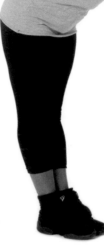

43

Twist back to face the front, bend your knees, and place your hands, palms flat, on your thighs, count 3

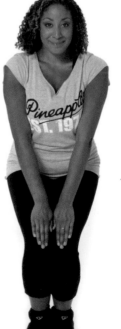

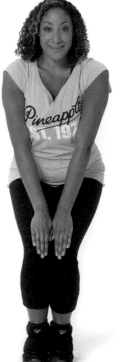

44

Twist your body to the left and, leaning forwards, push your arms out to the corner with flexed hands, both legs straight, count 4. Repeat steps 41 and 42, counts 5, 6

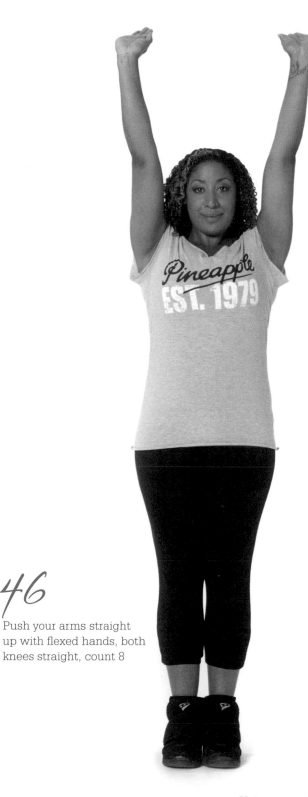

45

Twist back to face the front, bend your knees, and place your hands, palms flat, on your thighs, count 7

46

Push your arms straight up with flexed hands, both knees straight, count 8

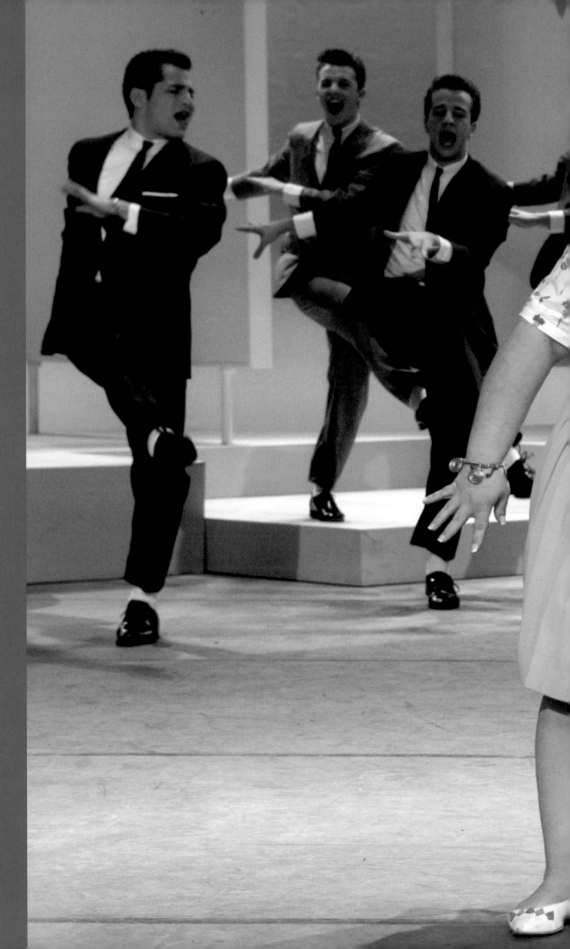

Tracy is the biggest and best dancer to ever perform on The Corny Collins Show. So no matter what your size, get up, join in and have fun

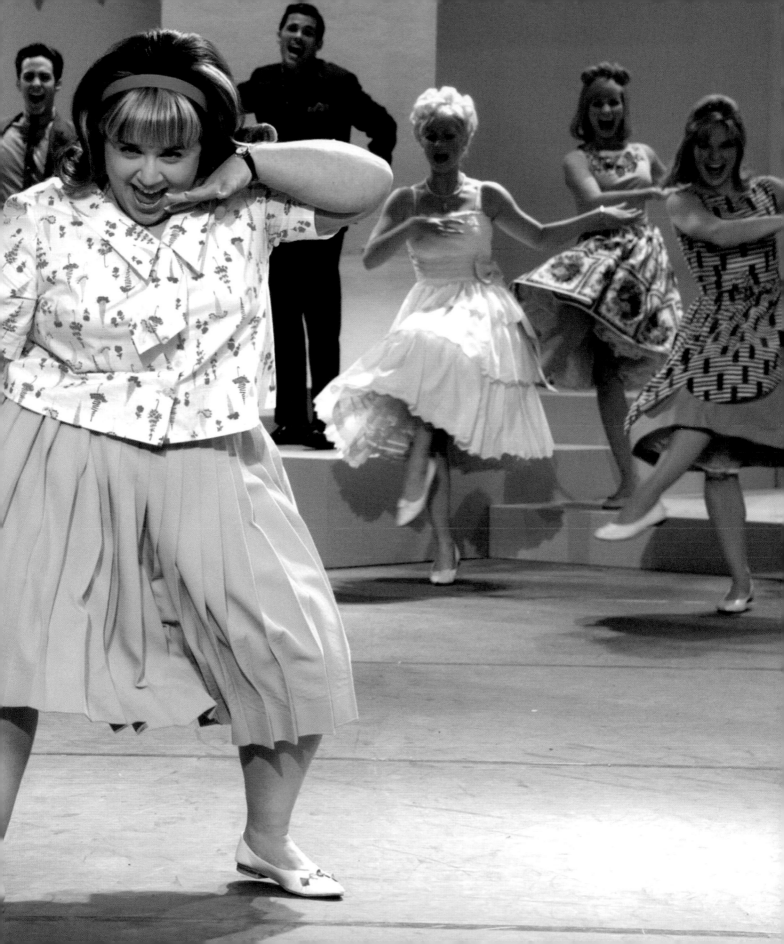

47

Step out to the side with your right foot, and bring both arms down to your sides, count 1

48

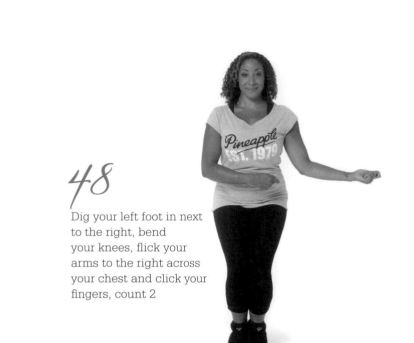

Dig your left foot in next to the right, bend your knees, flick your arms to the right across your chest and click your fingers, count 2

49

Step out to the side with your left foot, and bring both arms down to your sides, count 3

50

Dig your right foot in next to the left, bend your knees, flick your arms to the left across your chest and click your fingers, count 4

51

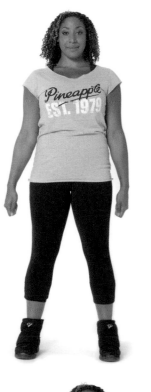

Step out to the side with your right foot, and bring both arms down to your sides, count 5

52

Bring your left foot in to join the right, circling your arms to the right, count 6

53

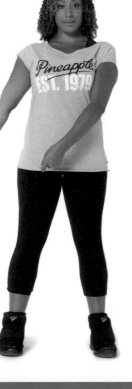

Step out to the side with your right foot, circling your arms down to the left, count 7

54

Dig your left foot in next to the right, bend your knees, flick your arms to the right across your chest and click your fingers, count 8

55

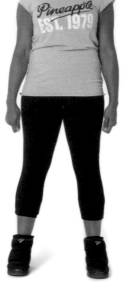

Step out to the side with your left foot, and bring both arms down to your sides, count 1

56

Dig your right foot in next to the left, bend your knees, flick your arms to the left across your chest and click your fingers, count 2

57

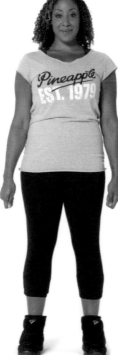

Step out to the side with your right foot, and bring both arms down to your sides, count 3

58

Dig your left foot in next to the right, bend your knees, flick your arms to the right across your chest and click your fingers, count 4

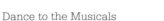

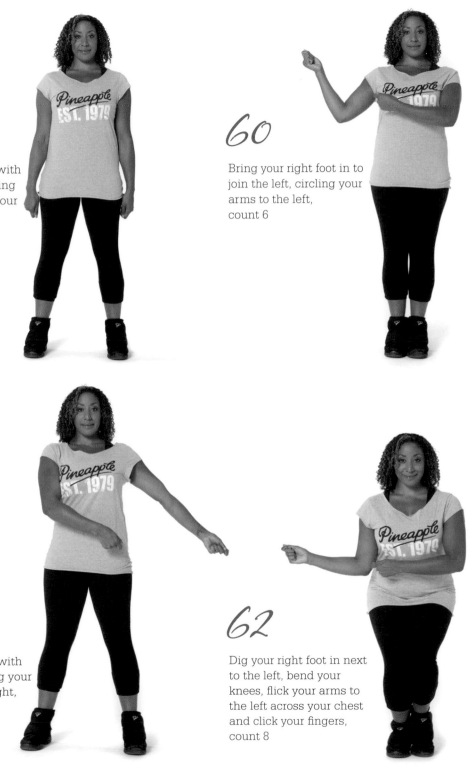

59

Step out to the side with your left foot, and bring both arms down to your sides, count 5

60

Bring your right foot in to join the left, circling your arms to the left, count 6

61

Step out to the side with your left foot, circling your arms down to the right, count 7

62

Dig your right foot in next to the left, bend your knees, flick your arms to the left across your chest and click your fingers, count 8

Twist your body to the left, flick your right foot forward and with your right arm make a semi-circle above your head from left to right, left arm parallel to the right leg, both hands in fists, count 1

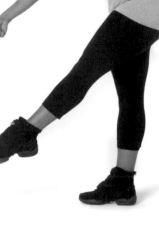

Bring your right leg back to join the left, bend your knees, and complete the semi-circle with your right arm, finishing with both arms next to each other, count 2.
Repeat steps 63 and 64 twice, counts 3, 4, 5, 6

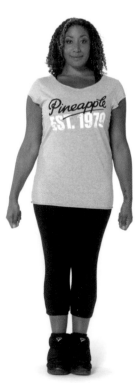

Jump landing with feet apart, face to the front, arms crossed, right over left, low in front of the body, hands in fists, count 7

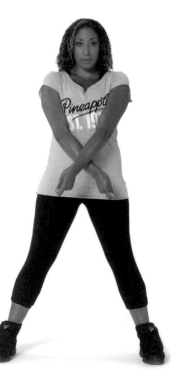

Jump landing with feet together, arms down by your sides, count 8

67

Twist your body to
the right, flick your
left foot forward
and with your left
arm make a semi-
circle above your
head from right
to left, right arm
parallel to the left
leg, both hands in
fists, count 1

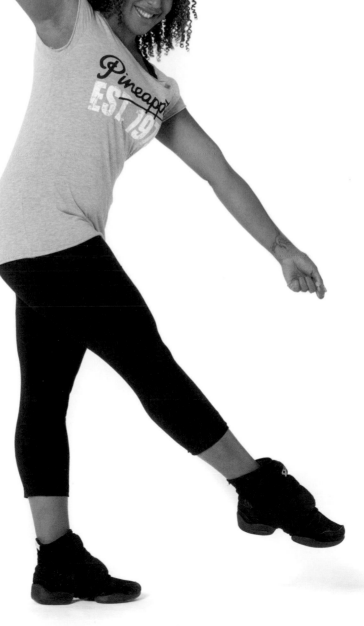

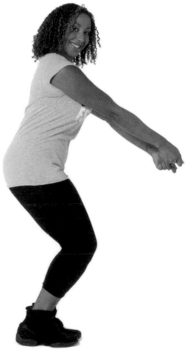

68

Bring your left leg back to join
the right, bend your knees, and
complete the semi-circle with
your left arm, finishing with
both arms next to each other,
count 2.
Repeat steps 67 and 68 twice,
counts 3, 4, 5, 6.
Repeat steps 65 and 66,
counts 7, 8

69

Flick your right leg out to front, bend your elbows, left arm forward, both hands in fists, count 1

70

Bring your right foot back to join the left, knees bent, right arm in line with the left, count 2.
Repeat steps 69 and 70 twice, counts 3, 4, 5, 6

71

Step out onto your right foot, left leg relaxed, both hands beside your face with palms facing the front, counts 7 hold 8

72

Flick your left leg out to front, bend your elbows, right arm forward, both hands in fists, count 1

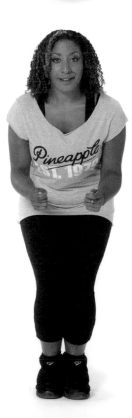

73

Bring your left foot back to join the right, knees bent, left arm in line with the left, count 2.
Repeat steps 72 and 73 twice, counts 3, 4, 5, 6

74

Step out onto your left foot, right leg relaxed, both hands beside your face with palms facing the front, counts 7 hold 8

75

Flick your right leg forward, left leg straight, left arm down, right arm raised at the back, both palms facing down, count 1

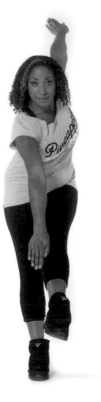

76

Bring your right foot back to join your left, bend your knees, left arm down by your side, right arm raised by the side of your head, count 2

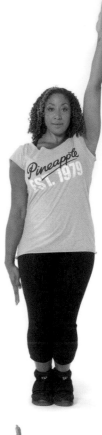

77

Flick your left leg forward, right leg straight, right arm down, left arm raised at the back, both palms facing down, count 3

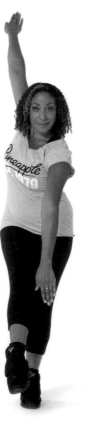

78

Bring your left foot back to join your right, bend your knees, right arm down by your side, left arm raised by the side of your head, count 4

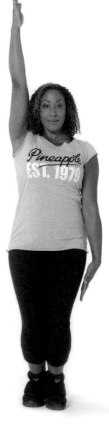

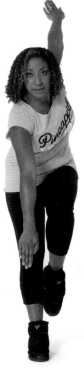

80

Bend your left leg, take your right leg in, keeping your arms in position, count 6

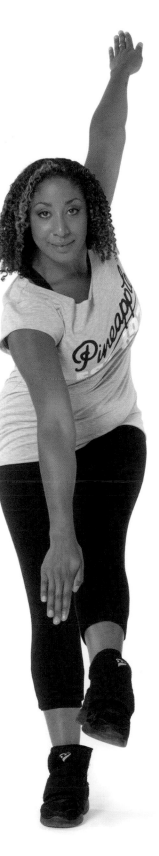

79

Flick your right leg forward, left leg straight, left arm down, right arm raised at the back, both palms facing down, count 5

81

Kick your right leg out, and stretch your knees, count 7

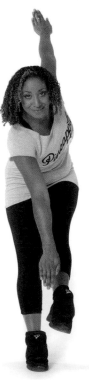

82

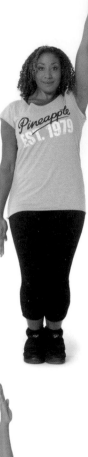

Bring your right foot back to join your left, bend your knees, left arm down by your side, right arm raised by the side of your head, count 8

83

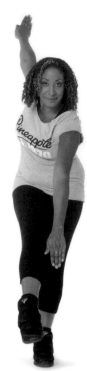

Flick your left leg forward, right leg straight, right arm down, left arm raised at the back, both palms facing down, count 1

84

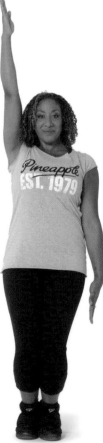

Bring your left foot back to join your right, bend your knees, right arm down by your side, left arm raised by the side of your head, count 2

85

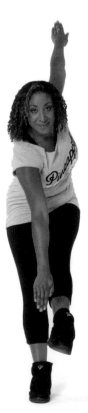

Flick your right leg forward, left leg straight, left arm down, right arm raised at the back, both palms facing down, count 3

86

Bring your right foot back to join your left, bend your knees, left arm down by your side, right arm raised by the side of your head, count 4

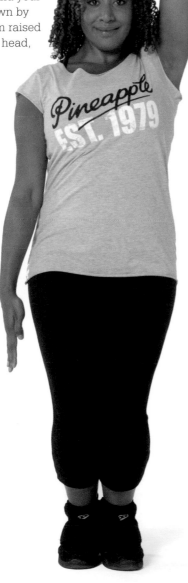

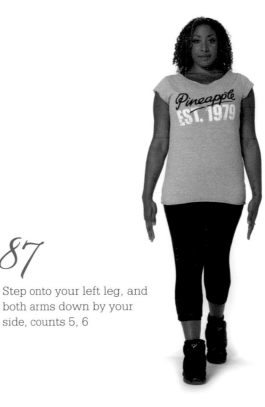

87

Step onto your left leg, and both arms down by your side, counts 5, 6

88

Bring your right foot to join your left, stretch your legs, hands beside face with palms facing out, counts 7 hold 8

As you build your stamina, repeat the entire routine from the beginning

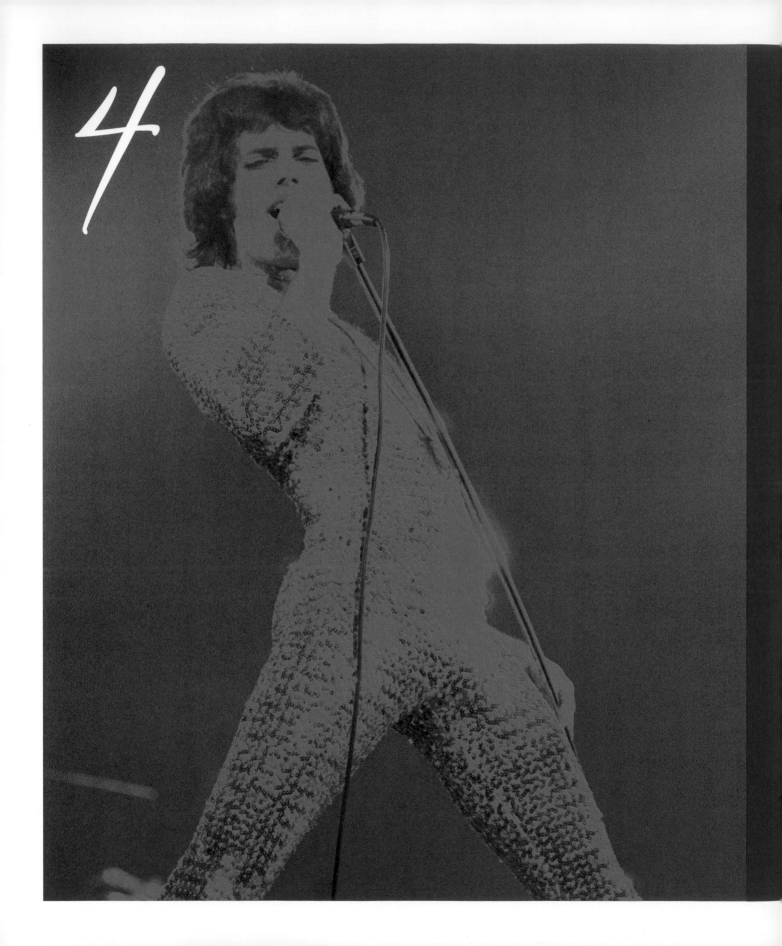

We Will Rock You

We Will Rock You

Written by Brian May

Creating the choreography for a new musical based on the music of Queen felt like a touch of magic. I'd worked with the glorious Freddie Mercury on videos for his solo album. 'I Was Born To Love You', filmed in what was then the derelict wasteland of Canary Wharf, had 360 marching girls in bizarre red plastic body suits. Freddie – wildly creative – was willing to try anything, however difficult. When I became part of his inner circle, we met at his extraordinary Kensington house, which was filled with octagonal mirrors. I will never forget trying to find the way out!

When I was asked to create the choreography for *We Will Rock You*, I was proud to work with the creative dream team of Ben Elton, Roger Taylor, Brian May, Mark Fisher and Willie Williams who were all funny, focused and exhausting. I had to create choreography which would serve as background to the story. Centre stage was Queen's music. Dance needed presence. It couldn't dominate. *We Will Rock You* opened in May to possibly the worst ever West End reviews. We thought it would close. Then, on 3 June, during the Party at the Palace to celebrate the Queen's Golden Jubilee, Brian played 'God Save the Queen' standing on the roof of Buckingham Palace. There was music from the show. Our cast, dressed in their amazing costumes, sang and danced their hearts out. Millions watched. Since then, *We Will Rock You* has sold out. I've worked on new productions in Australia, Las Vegas and Europe. Winner of the 2011 Olivier Audience Award, it's still the hottest ticket. This show is a survivor. My dance routine for 'We Will Rock You' is a punch in the air – brilliant for upper arms. As you jump and punch, feel the joy . . . You Rock!

My dance routine for 'We Will Rock You' starts with a punch in the air – brilliant for upper arms. As you jump and punch, feel the joy . . . You Rock!

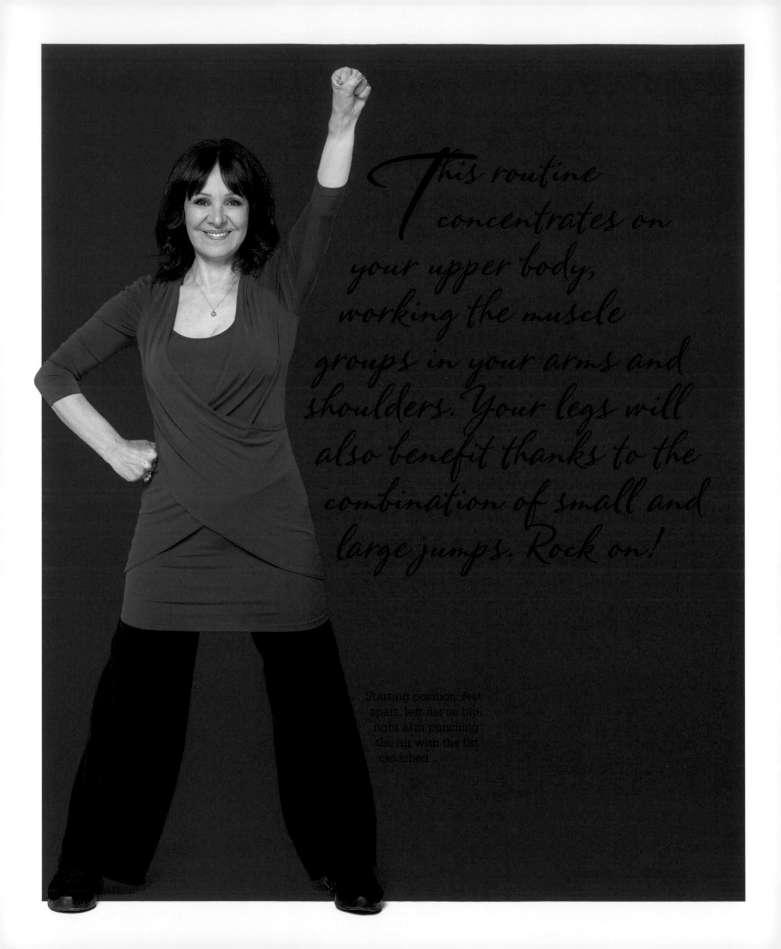

This routine concentrates on your upper body, working the muscle groups in your arms and shoulders. Your legs will also benefit thanks to the combination of small and large jumps. Rock on!

Starting position; feet apart, left fist on hip, right arm punching the air with the fist clenched

Part 1

1

Jump with your feet together. Clap twice above your head, counts 1, 'and'

2

Step forward with your left foot, and open your arms above your head, count 2

3

Clap twice above your head, with your feet together, counts 3 'and'

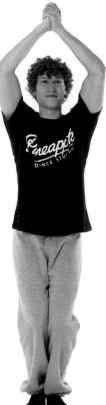

4

Step forward with your right foot, count 4. Repeat steps 1–4, counts 5, 'and' 6, 7, 'and' 8

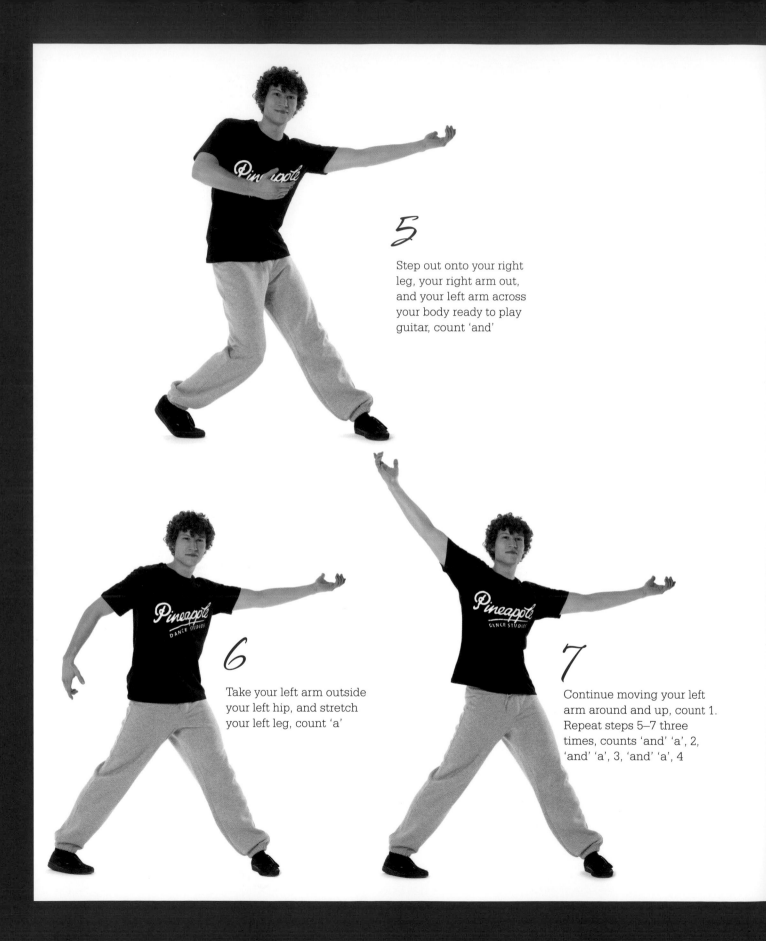

5

Step out onto your right leg, your right arm out, and your left arm across your body ready to play guitar, count 'and'

6

Take your left arm outside your left hip, and stretch your left leg, count 'a'

7

Continue moving your left arm around and up, count 1. Repeat steps 5–7 three times, counts 'and' 'a', 2, 'and' 'a', 3, 'and' 'a', 4

8

Lift your right leg, and 'play' the guitar with your left arm, count 5

9

Put your right leg down, and again 'play' guitar with your left arm, 6

10

Lift your right leg again, and 'play' the guitar with your left arm, count 7

11

Bring your feet together, and your arms down by the sides of your body, count 8.
Repeat steps 1–11

Part 2

12

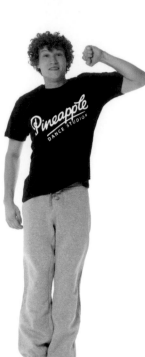

Jump with your feet together, bringing your right arm up, your hand in a fist beside your face, count 'and'

13

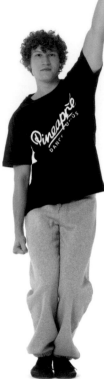

Land on both feet, punch your right arm above your head, with your hand still in a fist, count 1.
Repeat steps 12 and 13 three times, counts 'and', 2, 'and' 3, 'and' 4

14

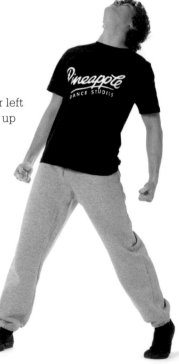

Step forward with your left leg, leaning your body up and back, count 'and'

15

Drop your body forward, with your arms behind you, hands still in fists, count 5.
Repeat steps 14 and 15, counts 'and' 6

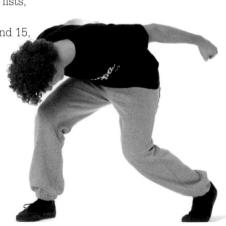

16

Step out to the opposite corner on your right foot, raising your body, and throwing your head back, count 'and'

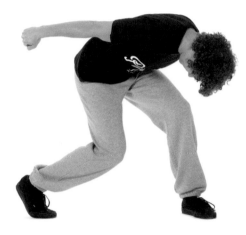

17

Drop your body forward, with your arms behind you, hands still in fists, count 7.
Repeat steps 16 and 17, counts 'and' 8

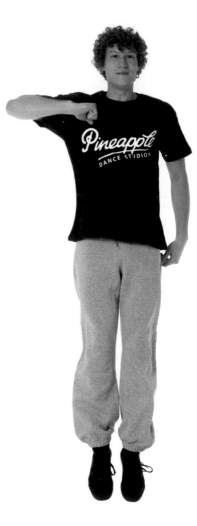

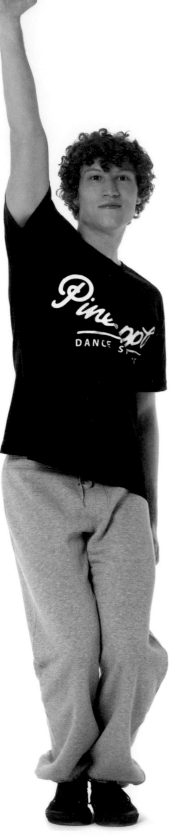

18

Jump with your feet together, bringing your left arm in to your chest, your hand in a fist, count 'and'

19

Land on both feet, stretch your left arm above your head, count 1.
Repeat steps 18 and 19 three times, counts 'and' 2, 'and' 3, 'and' 4

20

Step out with your right leg, raising your body and throwing back your head, count 'and'

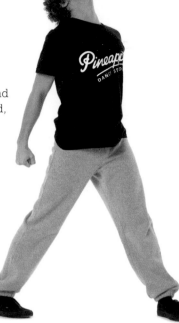

21

Drop your body forward, with your arms behind you, hands still in fists, count 5.
Repeat steps 20 and 21, counts 'and' 6

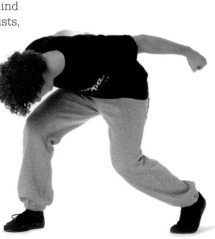

22

Step out to the opposite corner on your left foot, raising your body, and throwing your head back, count 'and'

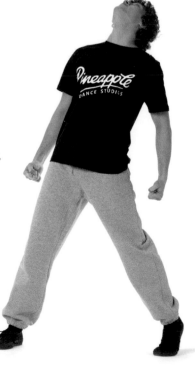

23

Drop your body forward, with your arms behind you, hands still in fists, count 7.
Repeat steps 22 and 23, counts 'and' 8

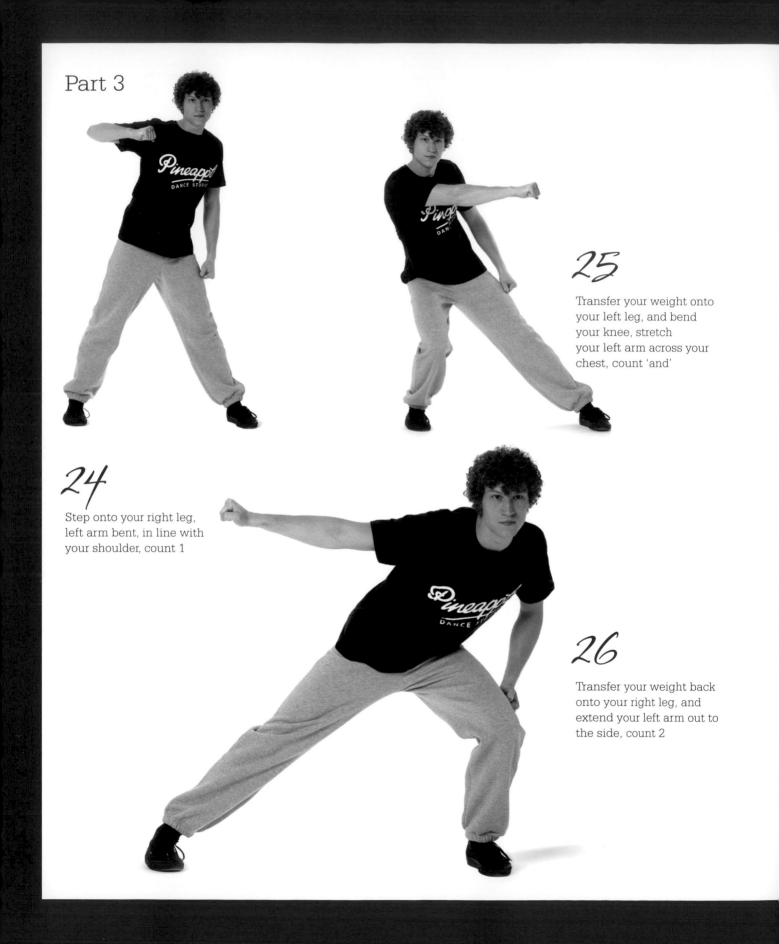

Part 3

25

Transfer your weight onto your left leg, and bend your knee, stretch your left arm across your chest, count 'and'

24

Step onto your right leg, left arm bent, in line with your shoulder, count 1

26

Transfer your weight back onto your right leg, and extend your left arm out to the side, count 2

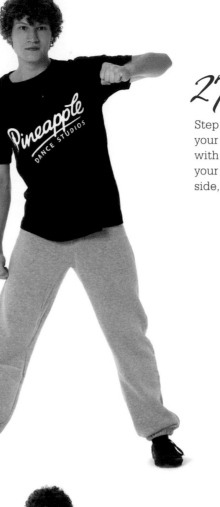

27

Step on your left leg, with your right arm bent in line with your shoulder, and your left arm down by your side, count 3

28

Transfer your weight onto your right leg, bend your knee and stretch your right arm across your chest, count 'and'

29

Transfer your weight back onto your left leg, and take your right arm out to the side, count 4

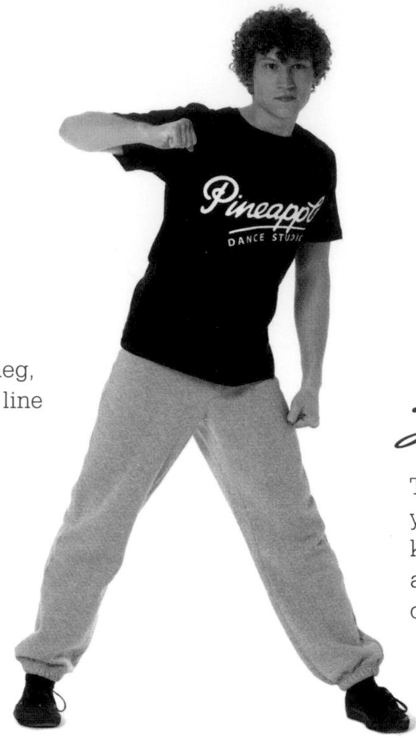

30

Step onto your right leg,
your left arm bent in line
with your shoulder,
count 5

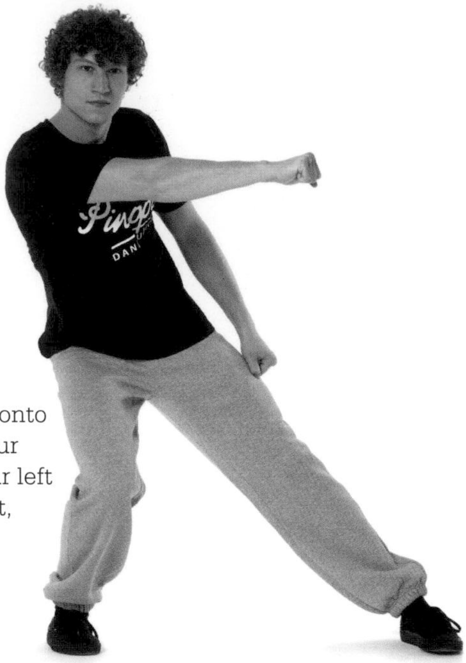

31

Transfer your weight onto
your left leg, bend your
knee, and stretch your left
arm across your chest,
count 'and'

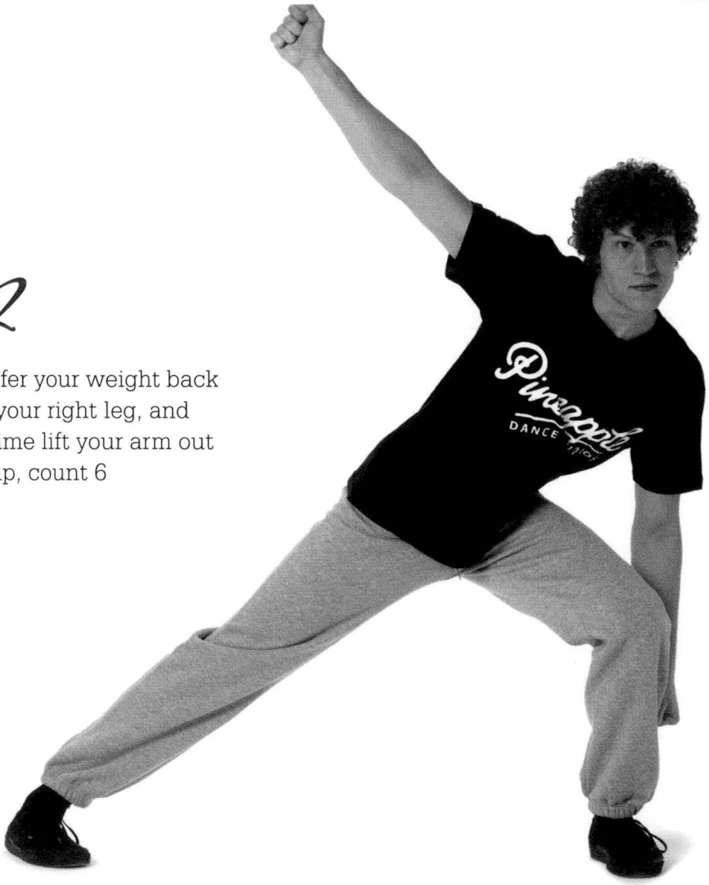

32

Transfer your weight back
onto your right leg, and
this time lift your arm out
and up, count 6

33

Step onto your left leg,
your right arm bent in line
with your shoulder,
count 7

34

Transfer your weight onto
your right leg, bend your
knee, and stretch your
right arm across your
chest, count 'and'

35

Transfer your weight back
onto your left leg, and lift
your arm out and up, count 8

36

Kick your right leg forward,
both arms to the side,
count 1

37

Step onto your right foot,
crossing over your left,
count 2

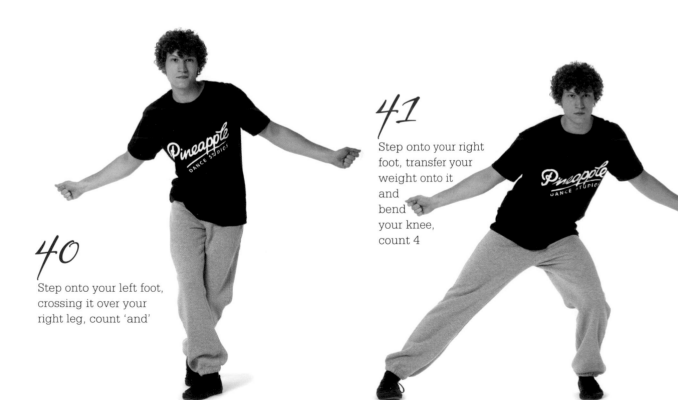

38

Step out to the side with your left foot, transfer your weight onto it and bend your knee, count 2

39

Kick your left leg forward, keeping your arms to the side, count 3

40

Step onto your left foot, crossing it over your right leg, count 'and'

41

Step onto your right foot, transfer your weight onto it and bend your knee, count 4

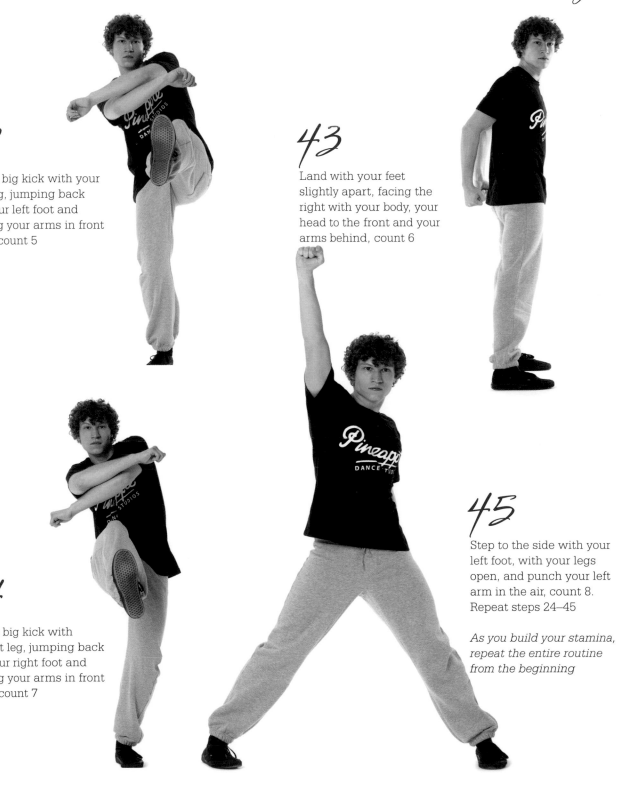

42
Make a big kick with your right leg, jumping back onto your left foot and crossing your arms in front of you, count 5

43
Land with your feet slightly apart, facing the right with your body, your head to the front and your arms behind, count 6

44
Make a big kick with your left leg, jumping back onto your right foot and crossing your arms in front of you, count 7

45
Step to the side with your left foot, with your legs open, and punch your left arm in the air, count 8. Repeat steps 24–45

As you build your stamina, repeat the entire routine from the beginning

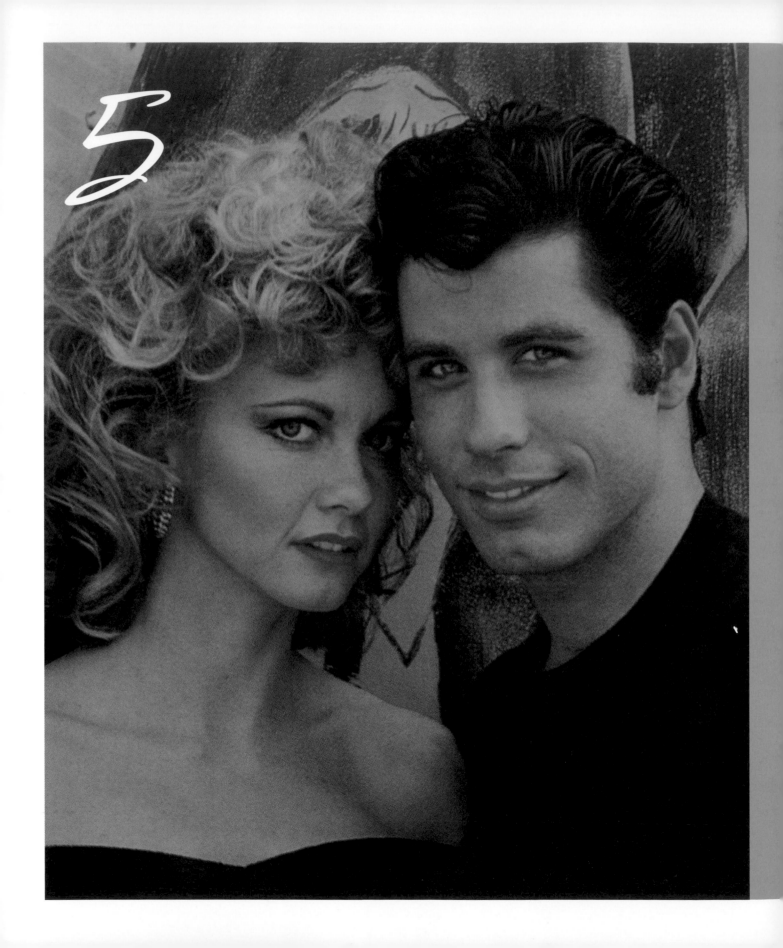

Grease

We Go Together

Written by Michael Gibson, Jim Jacobs and Warren Casey

It's hard to believe that it was a totally unknown Richard Gere who landed the star role as Danny in Grease when it first opened in London in 1973, after premiering on Broadway the previous year. It was a huge success and I couldn't wait to see it. The original stage musical had many songs but when Robert Stigwood decided to turn it into a film he asked the Bee Gees to write four new ones. These songs became the iconic tracks everyone knows, and the film became the highest-grossing movie musical ever made.

You won't need to put on your bobby socks or do the splits to dance 'We Go Together', but you'll feel the beat and work up a sweat with a smile on your face!

When the stage production opened at the Dominion Theatre in 2002 it was the first time the Bee Gees songs had been performed in the musical and it was then I came on board as the choreographer. A major headache was finding someone to play the bad boy role of Kenicke. One morning, Shane Ritchie turned up to audition. He explained that he'd had a nasty accident and had hurt his knee, and although it would be fine in two weeks' time, he couldn't risk dancing that day. When I asked what he could do, he reeled off every dance step imaginable and I thought, 'If he can do all that, he'll be fine'. But on the first day of rehearsals it was clear Shane didn't know his right from his left. He'd never taken a dance class in his life! I'd been completely taken in by Shane's charm. So I treated him like a naughty school boy, making him stay late for extra rehearsals, a tactic that paid off, as when the show opened he was fabulous.

You won't need to put on your bobby socks or do the splits to dance this routine, but you'll feel the beat and work up a sweat with a smile on your face. Dancing for joy doesn't get much better than this!

This is a fantastic cardiovascular routine that works all the major muscle groups in your legs and will also help to build strength in your shoulders and back to achieve a good body posture. Get on the dance floor and party!

Starting position: right arm crossed over the left in front of your chest, flexed hands with palms facing out to the sides

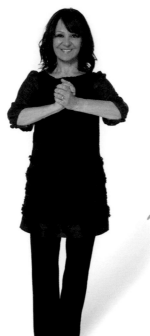

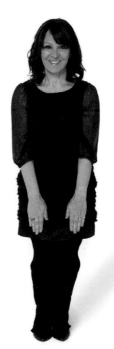

1

Feet together, clap hands
in front of your chest,
count 1

2

Smack your hands on your
thighs, and bend knees,
count 2

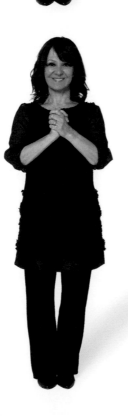

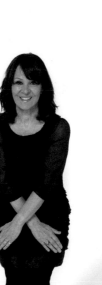

3

Clap your hands in front of
your chest, and straighten
both legs, count 3

4

Smack your hands on your
thighs, crossing your right
arm over the left, and bend
your knees, count 4.
Repeat steps 1 and 2,
counts 5, 6

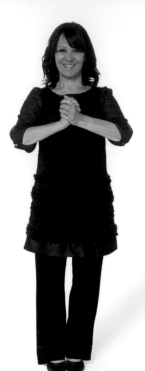

5

Clap your hands in front of your chest and straighten your legs, count 7

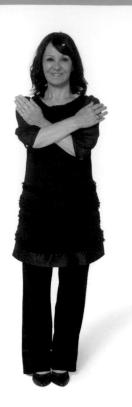

6

Cross your left arm over your right and place your hands on your shoulders, bend your knees, count 8

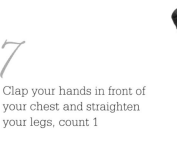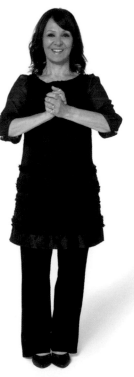

7

Clap your hands in front of your chest and straighten your legs, count 1

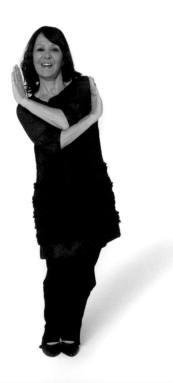

8

Cross your arms, right over left, in front of your chest, flexing your hands and bending your knees, count 2

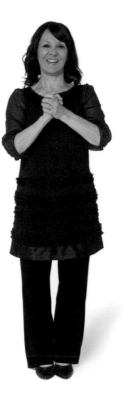

9

Clap your hands in front of
your chest and straighten
your legs, count 3

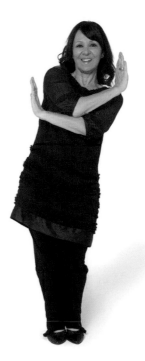

10

Cross your arms, left over
right, in front of your chest,
flexing your hands and
bending your knees,
count 4.
Repeat steps 7 and 8,
counts 5, 6

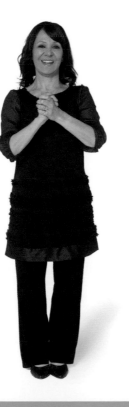

11

Clap your hands in front of
your chest and straighten
your legs, count 7

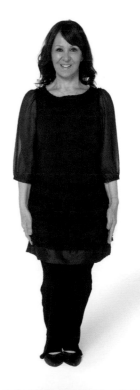

12

Lower your arms down by
your sides, count 8.
Repeat steps 1–12.

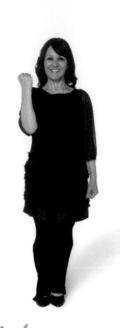

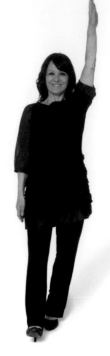

13

Put your right foot out to the front, heel on the floor, and raise your left arm, count 1

14

Bring your right foot back so your feet are together and pull your left arm down with a fist, count 'and'

15

Put your left foot out, heel on the floor, and raise your right arm, count 2

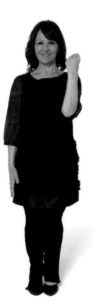

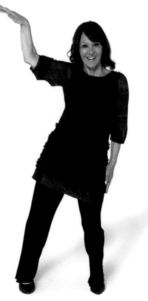

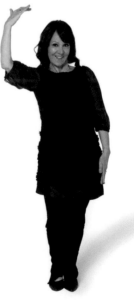

16

Bring your left foot back and pull your right arm down with a fist, count 'and'

17

Step out to side with your right leg, and flick your left hand out to side, count 3

18

Bring your left foot to join the right, and turn the left hand in, count 'and'

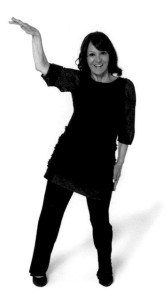

19

Step out to side with your right foot, and flick the left hand out, count 4

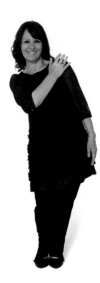

20

Bring the left foot to join the right and your left arm across your chest, count 'and'

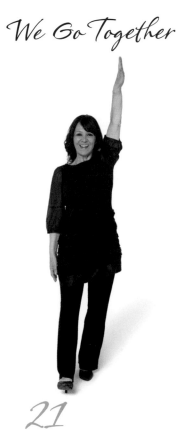

21

Put your left foot out to the front, heel on the floor and raise your right arm, count 5

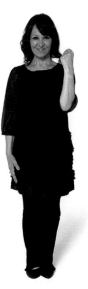

22

Bring your left foot back so your feet are together and pull your right arm down with a fist, count 'and'

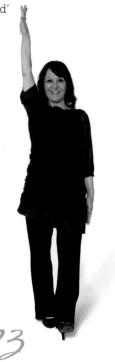

23

Put your right foot out to the front, heel on the floor, and raise your left arm, count 6

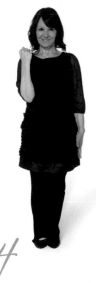

24

Bring your right foot back and pull your left arm down with a fist, count 'and'

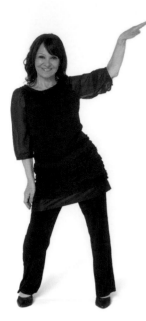

25

Step out to the side with your left leg, and flick your right hand out to the side, count 7

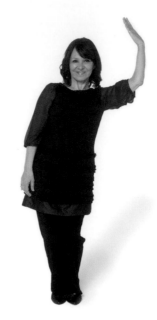

26

Bring your right foot to join the left, and turn your right hand in, count 'and'

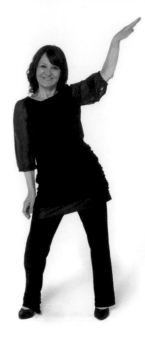

27

Step out to the side with your left foot, and flick your right hand out, count 8

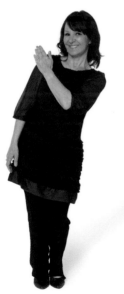

28

Bring your right foot to join your left, and your right arm across your chest, count 'and'

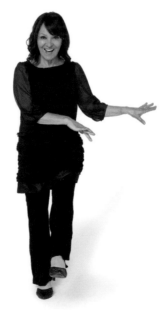

29

Kick your right leg forward, flicking both hands across your body to the right, count 1

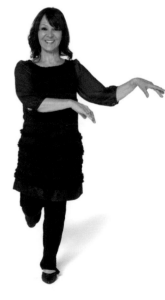

30

Drop onto your right leg, and lift your left foot behind you, count 'and'

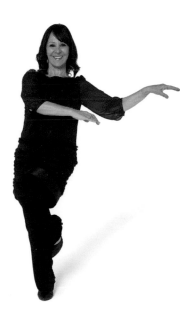

31

Kick your left leg forward, and flick your hands to the left, count 2

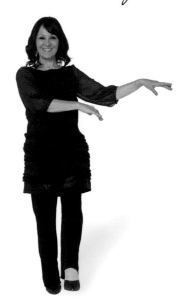

32

Drop onto your left leg and lift your right foot behind you, count 'and'

33

Kick your right leg forward, and flick your hands to the right, count 3

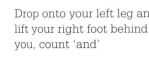

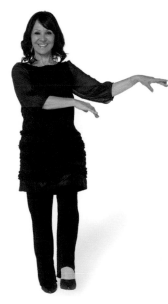

34

Bend your left knee, bring your right foot in to your left calf, count 'and'

35

Kick your right leg forward, count 4

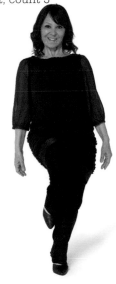

36

Drop onto your right leg, bring your left foot in to your calf, and drop arms to your sides, count 'and'

37

Kick your left leg forward, and flick your hands to the left, count 5

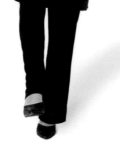

38

Drop onto your left leg and lift your right foot behind you, count 'and'

39

Kick your right leg forward and flick your hands to the right, count 6

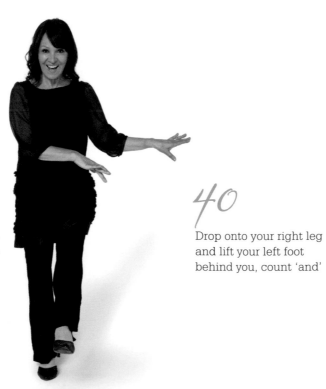

40

Drop onto your right leg and lift your left foot behind you, count 'and'

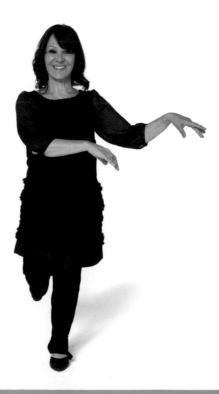

41

Kick your left leg forward and flick your hands to the left, count 7

42

Bend your right knee, and bring your left leg in to your right calf, count 'and'

43

Kick your left leg forward, count 8

44

Drop onto your left leg, raise your right foot behind you, and drop your arms to your sides, count 'and'. Repeat steps 13–44

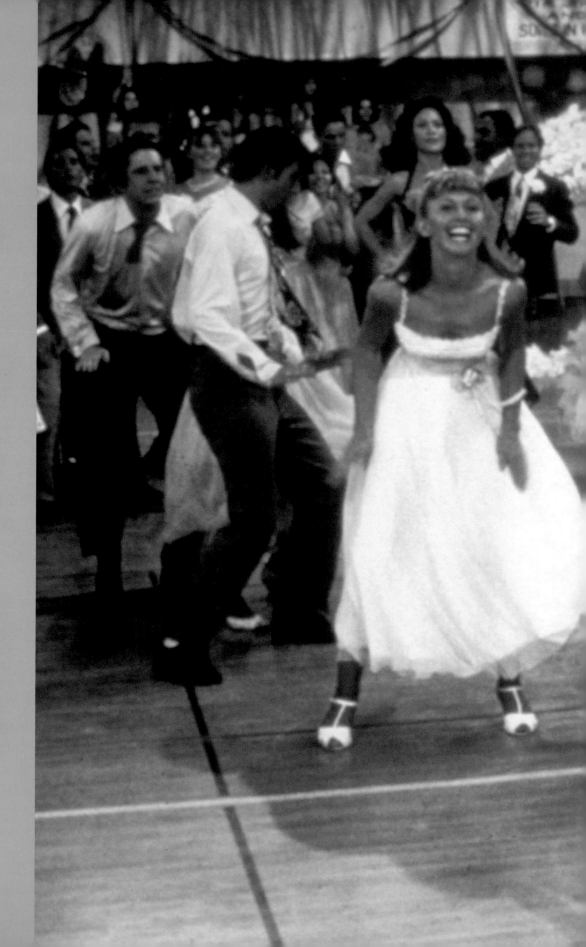

Who doesn't remember the
High School Hop and Danny
and Sandy's 'Born to Hand
Jive'? John Travolta looks so
cool – as always

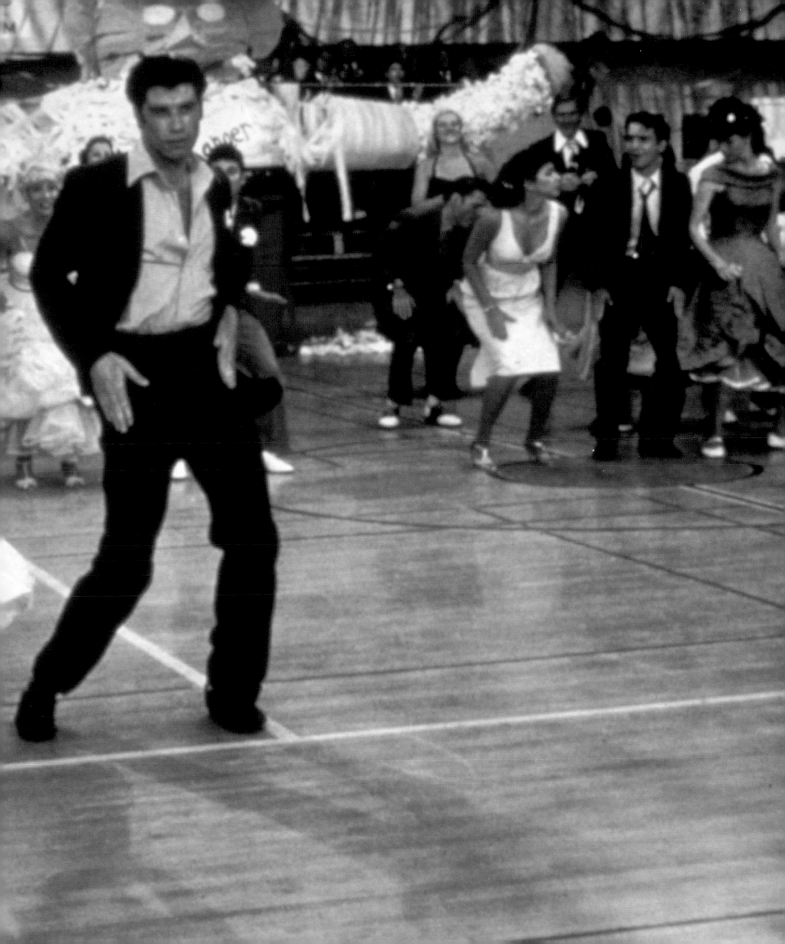

45

Jump to the left, and land with your feet together, knees slightly bent, and your right arm raised, count 1

46

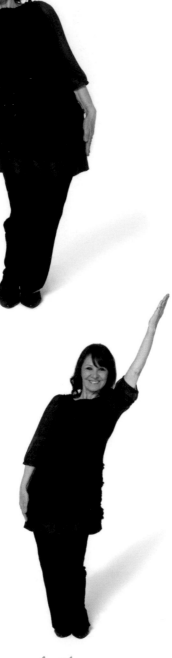

Jump to the right, land with your feet together, knees slightly bent, and your left arm raised, count 2

47

Jump to the left, feet together, knees slightly bent, and your right arm raised, count 3

48

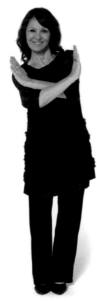

Cross your arms, left over right, in front of your chest, count 'and'

49

Raise your right arm, left down by your side, count 4

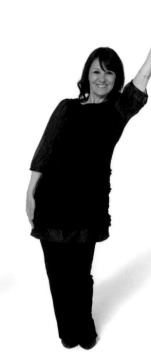

52

Jump to the right, feet together, knees slightly bent, and your left arm raised, count 7

50

Jump to the right, feet together, knees slightly bent, and your left arm raised, count 5

51

Jump to the left, feet together, knees slightly bent, and your right arm raised, count 6

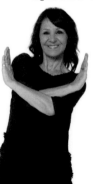

53

Cross your arms, right over left, in front of your chest, count 'and'

54

Raise your right arm, left down by your side, count 8

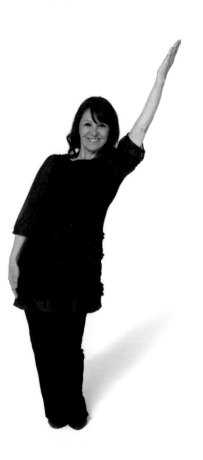

55

Step out with your right foot, right knee bent, left arm out to the side, elbow bent, and your hand with fingers splayed in front of your waist, count 1

56

Step onto your left foot and change arms so your right arm is out to the side, elbow bent, and your right hand with fingers splayed is in front of your waist, count 2

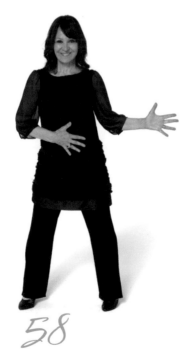

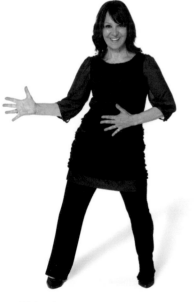

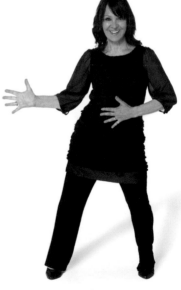

57

Step out with your right foot, right knee bent, left arm out to the side, elbow bent, and your hand with fingers splayed in front of your waist, count 3

58

Switch arms, twisting your body, with your heels off the floor and straight knees, to the left, count 'and'

59

Twist your legs back to face the front, switching your arms, count 4

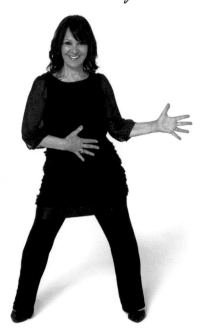

60

Step onto your left foot and change arms so your right arm is out to the side, elbow bent, and your right hand with fingers splayed is in front of your waist, count 5

61

Step onto your right foot, and switch your arms so the left hand is in front of your waist, count 6

62

Step onto your left foot and switch arms so your right hand is in front of your waist, count 7

63

Switch arms again, twisting your body with your heels off the floor and straight knees, to the right corner, count 'and'

64

Twist your legs back to face the front, switching your arms so your right hand is in front of your waist, count 8.
Repeat steps 45–64

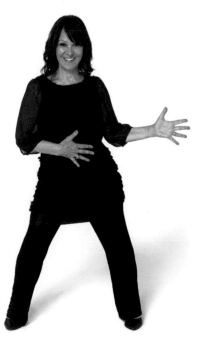

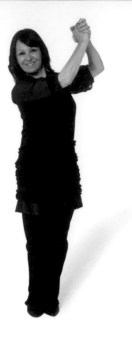

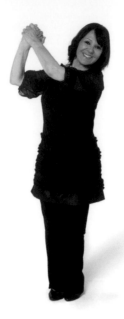

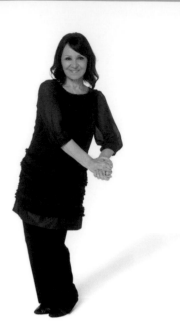

65

Jump to the right, land with your feet together, count 1, clap hands up to the right, count 'and'

66

Jump to the left, land with your feet together, count 2, clap hands up to the left, count 'and'

67

Jump to the right, count 3, clap hands down to the right, count 'and'

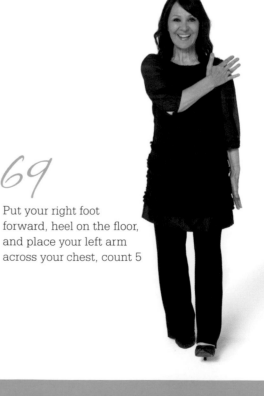

68

Jump to the left, count 4, clap hands down to the left, count 'and'

69

Put your right foot forward, heel on the floor, and place your left arm across your chest, count 5

70

Bring your right foot to join
the left, bend your knees,
and flick your left hand
out, count 'and'

71

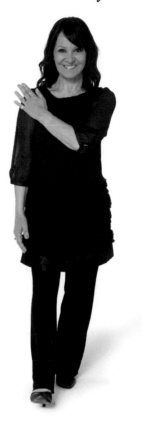

Put your left foot forward,
heel on the floor, and place
your right arm across your
chest, count 6

72

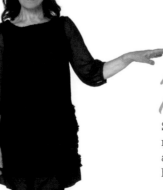

Bring your left foot to
join your right, bend your
knees, and flick your right
hand out to the side,
count 'and'

73

Step to the side on your
right foot, circling your left
arm out to the side, your
hand in a fist, count 7

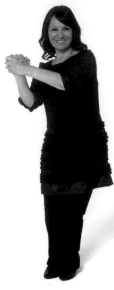

 74

Jump to the left with feet together, count 8, clap your hands by your left shoulder, count 'and'

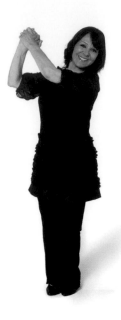

 75

Jump to the left, count 1, clap your hands to the left up high, count 'and'

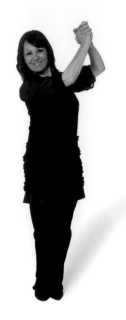

76

Jump to the right, count 2, clap your hands to the right up high, count 'and'

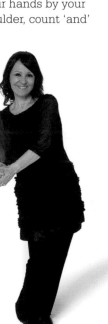

77

Jump to the left, count 3, clap your hands low to the left, count 'and'

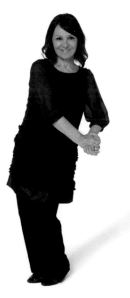

 78

Jump to the right, count 4, clap your hands low to the right, count 'and'

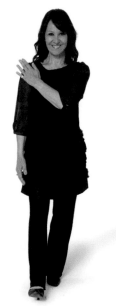

 79

Put your left foot forward, heel on the floor, and place your right arm across your chest, count 5

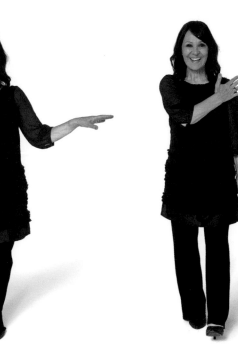

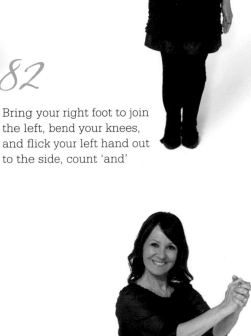

82

Bring your right foot to join the left, bend your knees, and flick your left hand out to the side, count 'and'

80

Bring your left foot to join the right, bend your knees, and flick your right hand out, count 'and'

81

Put your right foot forward, heel on the floor, and place your left arm across your chest, count 6

83

Step to the side onto your left foot, circling your right arm out to the side, with your hand as a fist, count 7

84

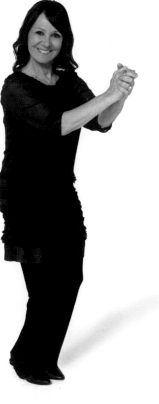

Jump with your feet together, count 8, clap your hands in front of your chest, count 'and'

As your stamina builds, repeat the entire routine from the beginning

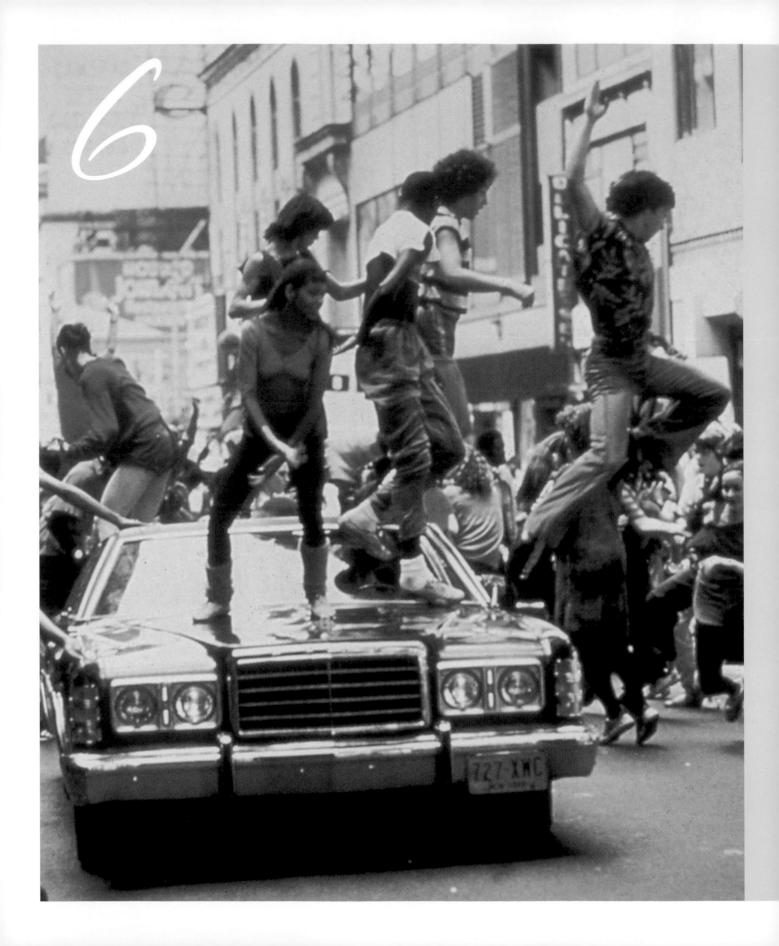

Fame

Fame

Written by Michael Gore and Dean Pitchford

> *It's music that makes you want to dance and will lift your spirits at any time of day or night. It's easy, it's fun, and will do your whole body good*

Fame is one of the most exciting dance films ever! In my opinion, the music and the dance routines are made for each other. It's virtually impossible to see, listen and watch without wanting to get up and join in! The choreography for the big 'Fame' number looks very free and improvised. The genius of it, however, was that this couldn't have been further from the truth. Although it has the appearance of an incredible free-for-all, it was dance built step by step, with the camera specifically placed for each shot – a long, painstaking process of which the audience is totally unaware. I was lucky enough to work with Antonia Franceschi who played Hilary, the ballerina in the film, and she truly was a star dancer.

The 1982 spin-off TV musical-drama series was also a massive hit everywhere. The choreography for the TV series was done by Debbie Allen, who also played Lydia, the dance teacher. In character, she approached teaching dance as a physical art form, which is exactly how I work. Lydia is a tough, no-nonsense teacher. She knows that dance has to be a passion and that it's also painful and hard work. Above all, she knows that a dancer has to be disciplined, and want to dance more than anything else. As a teacher, that's what I demand. I watched her in the TV series, thinking, 'This could be me!'

The title song, 'Fame', is up-tempo and has a driving beat that makes you want to dance and will lift your spirits at any time of day or night. The routine is easy, it's fun, it's addictive, and it will do your whole body good. What's not to like?

This routine is an all-over body workout that requires grace and style. Pull it in and pull it up!

Starting position: feet apart, right fist on right hip, left hand pointing down with left arm forward, left knee bent and prepare to transfer your weight onto the left foot

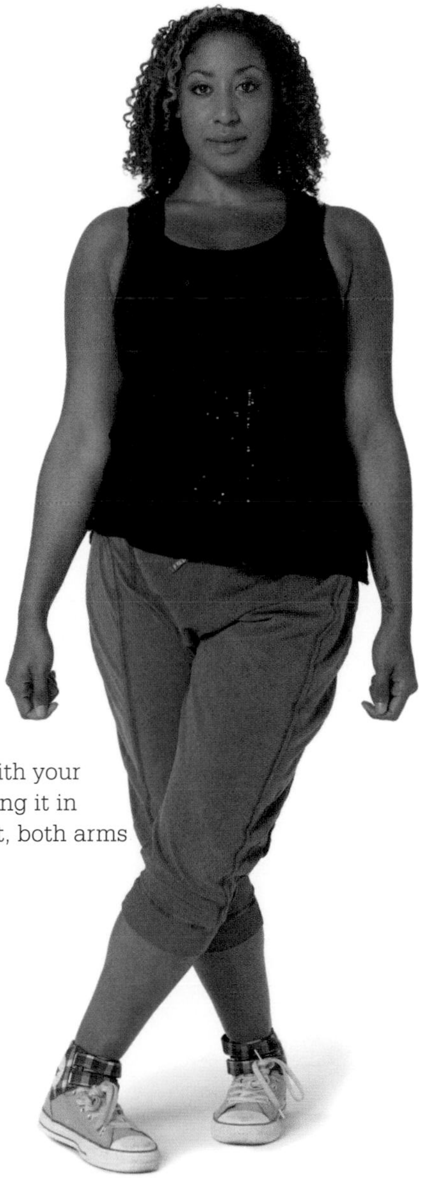

1

Step forward with your
right foot crossing it in
front of your left, both arms
down, count 1

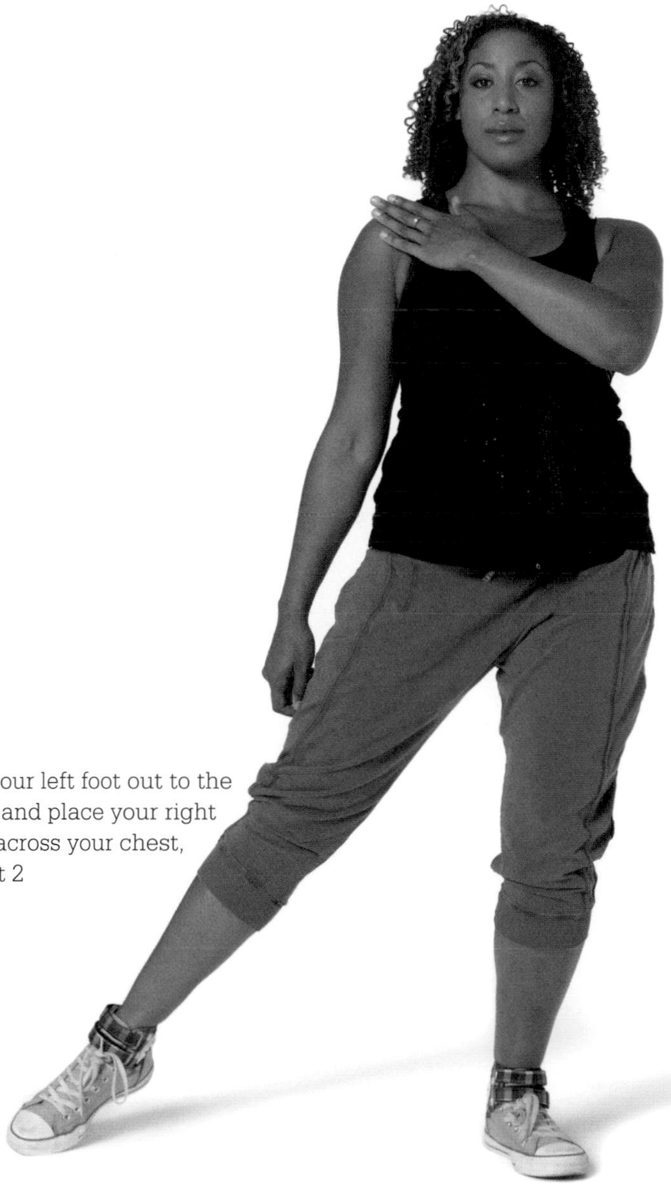

2

Put your left foot out to the
side, and place your right
arm across your chest,
count 2

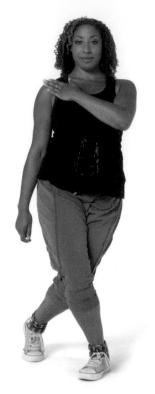

Step forward with your left foot, crossing it in front of your right, right arm still across your chest, count 3

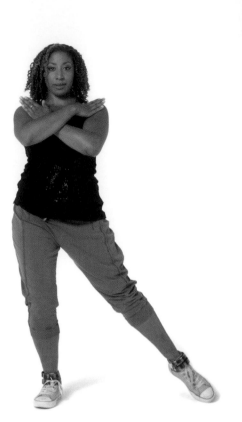

4

Put your right foot out to the side, and place your left arm across your chest on top of your right, count 4

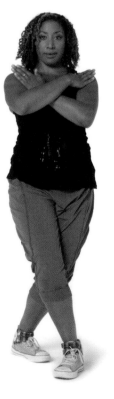

5

Step back with your right foot crossing it behind your left, arms still crossed, count 5

6

Put your left leg out to the side, and bring your left arm down to side, count 6

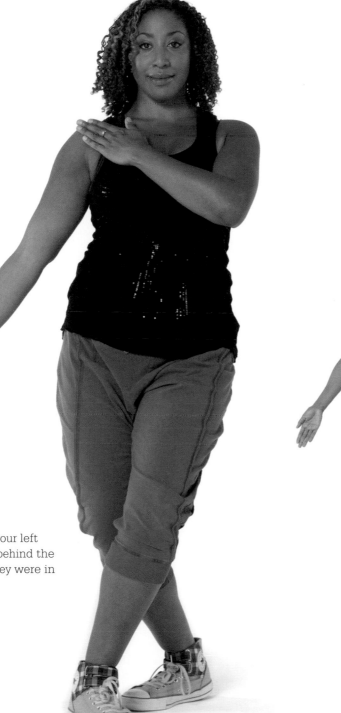

7

Step back onto your left foot, crossing it behind the right, arms as they were in step 6, count 7

8

Put your right leg out to the side, and bring your right arm down to side, count 8

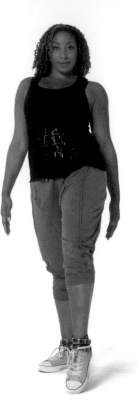

Touch your right foot forward, keeping your heel off the floor, and pushing your right hip up, arms down by your sides, count 1

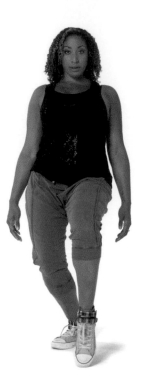

10

Bend both your knees, keeping your right hip down, count 2

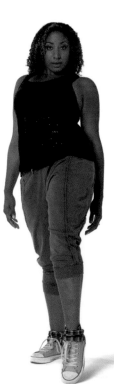

11

Push your right hip up, and stretch your left leg, count 3

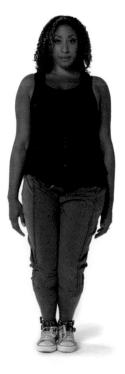

12

Bring your right foot in, so your feet are together, and your knees bent, count 4

13

Touch your left foot forward, keeping your heel off the floor, and pushing your left hip up, count 5

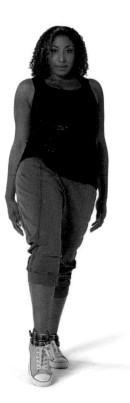

14

Bend both your knees, and push your left hip down, count 6

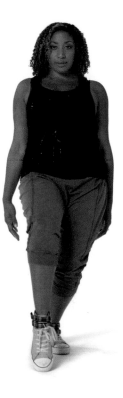

15

Push your left hip up, and stretch your right leg, count 7

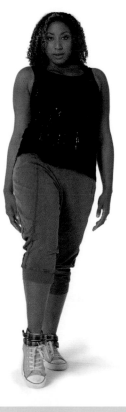

16

Bring your left foot in, so your feet are together, knees bent, count 8

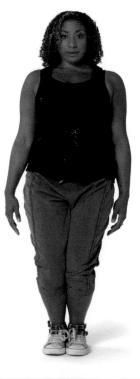

17

Step onto your right foot, slightly lifting your left foot off the floor, and bend your arms making fists next to your cheeks, count 'and'

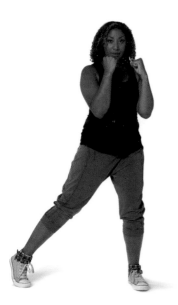

18

Step to the side onto the ball of your left foot, keeping your arms in position, count 'a'

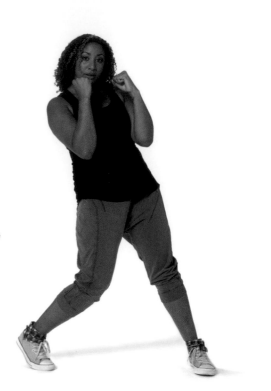

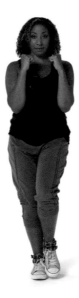

19

Step back onto your right foot, count 1

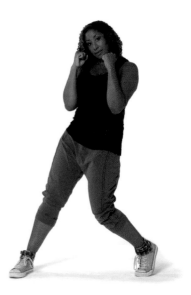

20

Step onto your left foot, slightly lifting your right foot off the floor, keeping your arms bent with fists next to your cheeks, count 'and'

21

Step to the side onto the ball of your right foot, keeping your arms in position, count 'a'

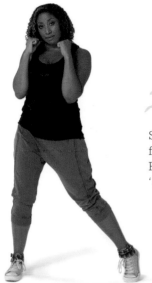

22

Step back onto your left
foot, count 2.
Repeat steps 17–22, counts
'and', 'a', 3, 'and', 'a', 4

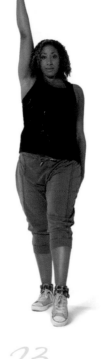

23

Place your right foot
forward, both legs straight,
and raise your left arm
keeping your hand open,
count 5

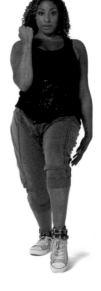

24

Bend both your knees, and
pull your left arm down
with a fist, count 6

25

Place your left foot
forward, both legs straight,
and raise your right arm
keeping your hand open,
count 7

26

Bring your left leg next to
your right, and pull your
right arm down, count 8.
Repeat steps 17–26, counts
'and', 'a', 1, 'and', 'a', 2,
'and', 'a', 3, 'and', 'a', 4, 5,
6, 7, 8.
Repeat steps 1–26

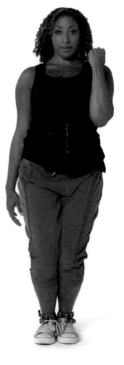

Put your right leg out to
the side, lifting your heel
off the floor, keeping both
hands on your thighs,
but with the left arm
bent, and your right arm
stretched, count 1

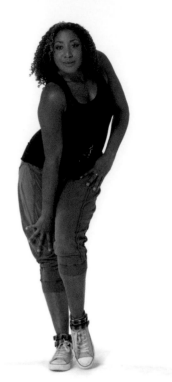

Bring your right foot to join
the left, keeping your heel
off the floor, both knees
bent, left arm stretched,
and right arm bent,
count 2

Open your right knee out
to the side, turn your head
to the right, bend your left
arm and stretch the right,
count 3

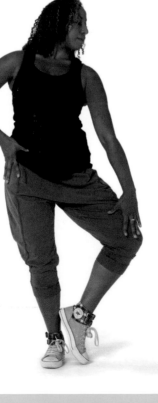

Bring your right knee
to the front, keeping it
bent, bend your right
arm, and stretch out the
left, count 4.
Repeat steps 27–30, counts
5, 6, 7, 8

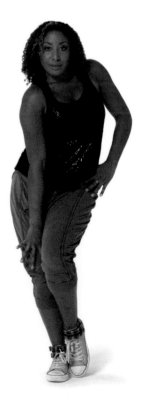

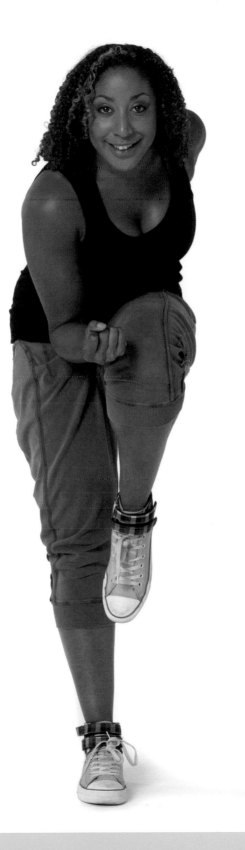

31

Lift your right knee and point your foot towards the floor, straighten your left leg, bend your left arm clicking your fingers, and keep your right arm beside your body, count 1

32

Step onto your right leg, so your left leg is to the side, keeping your right hand by your body and your left arm down across your body, count 2

33

Lift your left knee, keeping your right leg straight, click the fingers of your right hand, keeping your left arm by your body, count 3

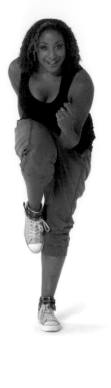

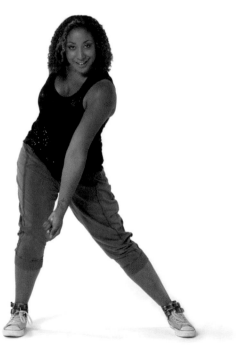

34

Step onto your left leg, bringing your right arm down across your body, count 4

35

Make a little kick forwards with your right foot, raising both arms to the side, count 5

36

Drop onto your right foot, bend both knees, bringing both arms down with flexed hands, count 6

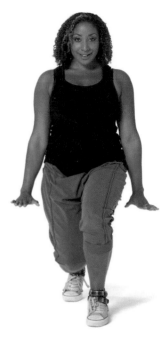

37

Kick with your right foot, both arms down and back, clicking your fingers, upper body leaning back, count 7

38

Bring your right foot to join the left, arms down by your sides, count 8. Repeat steps 27–38.

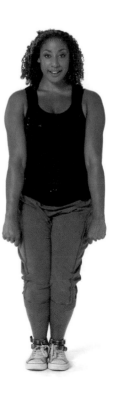

39

Touch your right heel to the floor in front of you, bend your left leg, and with straight arms and flexed hands, push down with your right arm, count 1

40

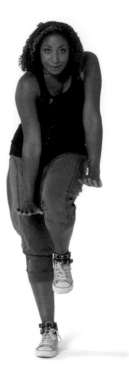

Lift your right heel off the floor, bend your right knee, and push down with your left arm, count 2. Repeat steps 39 and 40, counts 3, 4

41

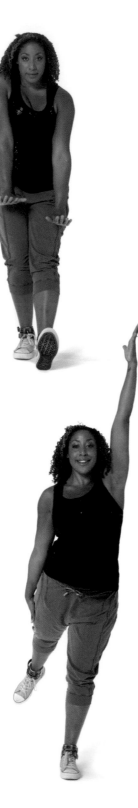

Jump onto your right leg, throwing your left leg back and off the floor, raising your right arm and lowering your left, and keeping your palms flat, count 5

42

Bend your right leg, bring your left knee and your arms into your chest, making fists with your hands, count 6

43

Jump onto your left leg, and throw your right leg back and off the floor, and raise your left arm up, count 7

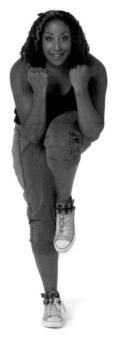

44

Bend your left leg, bring your right knee and your arms into your chest, making fists with your hands, count 8

45

Step out to the side with your right foot, circling your arms down and up with bent elbows, keeping your hands as fists, count 1

46

Transfer your weight onto your right foot, continuing to circle your arms up and into your chest, count 'and'

47

Step so your left foot crosses behind the right, circling your arms down and up with bent elbows, count 2

48

Step out to the side with your left leg, and circle your arms out and down, count 3

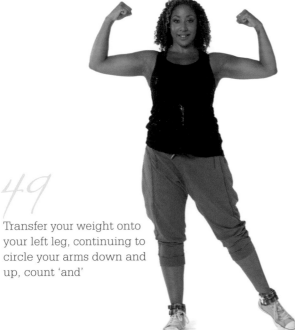

49

Transfer your weight onto your left leg, continuing to circle your arms down and up, count 'and'

50

Step so your right foot crosses behind the left, bending both knees, continuing to circle your arms, finishing in a clap with straight arms at the front, count 4

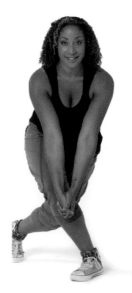

51

Step out onto your right foot, feet apart, raise your left arm up and across, keeping your right arm down, and look up to your left hand, counts 5, hold 6

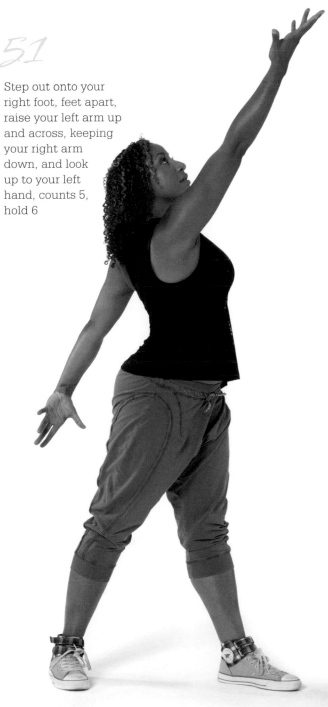

52

Step onto your left foot, feet apart, bring your left arm down and your right arm down and across, and look down to your right hand, count 7

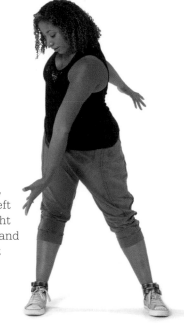

53

Bring your right foot to join your left, both arms down to your sides, and look to the front, count 8. Repeat steps 39–53

As you build your stamina, repeat the entire routine from the beginning

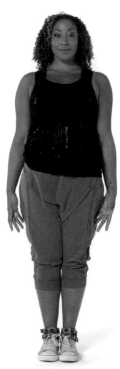

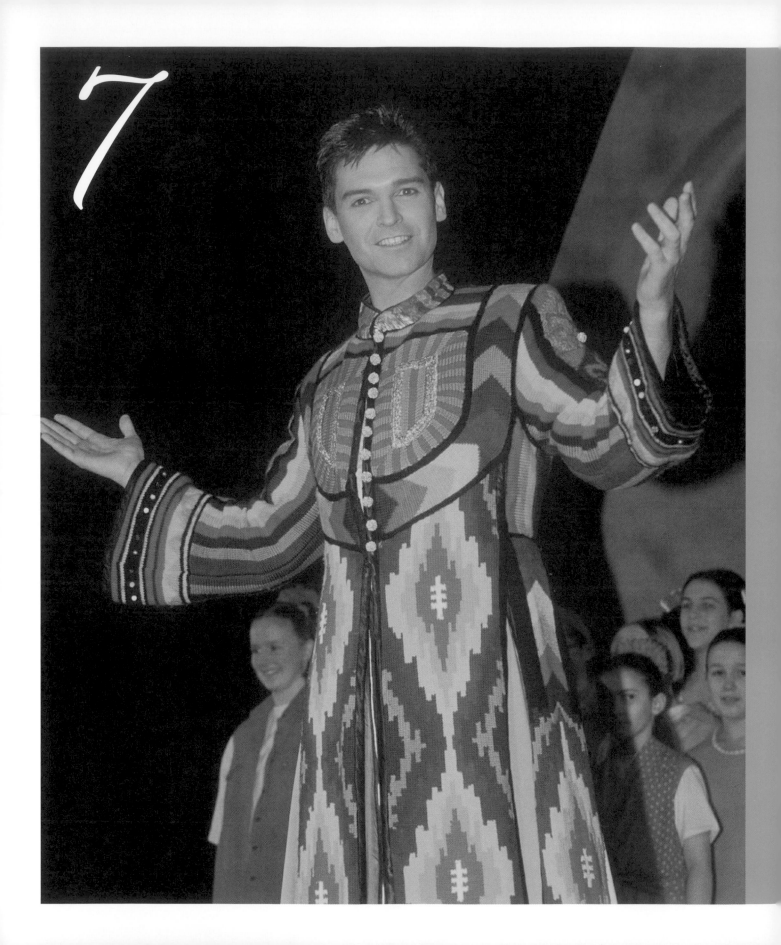

Joseph

Go Go Go Joseph

Written by Andrew Lloyd Webber and Tim Rice

> 'Go Go Go Joseph' throws in lots of leg and arm work – everyone is going to be able to do these moves and feel like they're doing a full body workout

Joseph and the Amazing Technicolor Dreamcoat was originally commissioned from Andrew Lloyd Webber and Tim Rice as a 15-minute 'pop cantata' by Alan Doggett, head of Colet Court, London, for the preparatory school choir to sing at their Easter concert on 1 March 1968. Productions have been running somewhere in the world ever since. When Donny Osmond played Joseph in Canada, for example, he took the country by storm and became the ultimate musical theatre performer.

I was one of the names discussed as a potential choreographer of the 1991 revival of *Joseph*. I didn't get the job, but that didn't stop me screaming and shouting for Jason Donovan with the rest of the ecstatic first night audience. I did, however, choreograph the US touring show starring Patrick Cassidy, which opened in Kentucky and had former cheerleaders as cast members who could do phenomenal, hair-raising tricks on stage. The boys tossed the girls in the air, they'd then do triple turns, before landing back in the boys' arms. The audiences used to stand and cheer!

'Go Go Go Joseph' has a real 60s feel. It was a time when everyone went out to clubs and dance halls and the music was easy to bounce around to. My routine reflects this with lots of iconic leg and arm moves – everyone is going to be able to do these 60s moves and feel like they're doing a full body workout.

This routine will build your stamina while you're having fun. Your fitness level, coordination and rhythm skills will be improved by mastering this choreography. Stay loose and feel the bounce!

Starting position: stand with your feet apart, lift the elbows and flex your wrists and hands

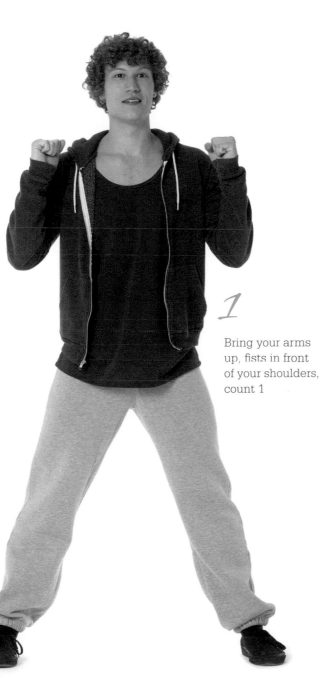

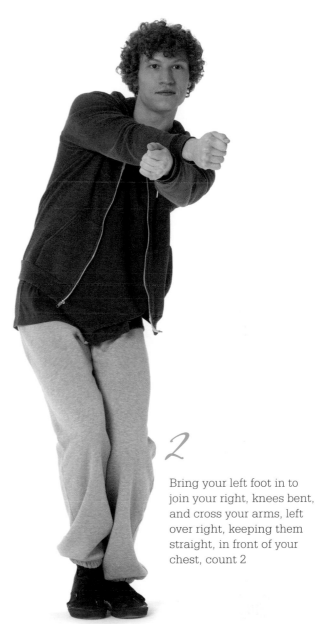

1

Bring your arms up, fists in front of your shoulders, count 1

2

Bring your left foot in to join your right, knees bent, and cross your arms, left over right, keeping them straight, in front of your chest, count 2

3

Step out with your left foot, fists in front of your shoulders, count 3

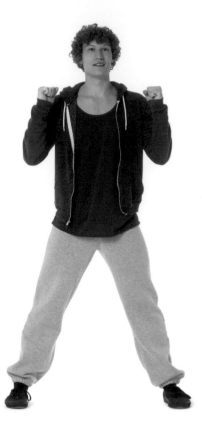

4

Bring your right foot to join the left, knees bent, and cross your arms, left over right, keeping them straight, in front of your chest, count 4

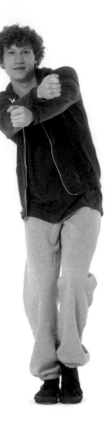

5

Step out with your right foot, fists in front of your shoulders, count 5

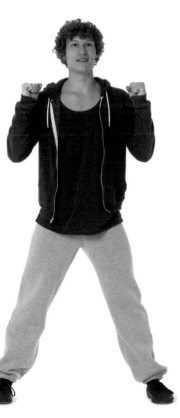

6

Bring your left foot to join the right, knees bent, and cross your arms, left over right, keeping them straight, in front of your chest, count 6

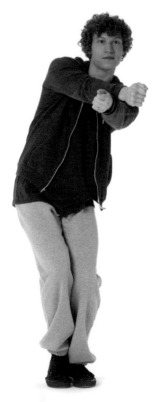

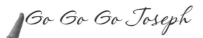

7

Jump, feet apart, and raise both arms, palms facing out, count 7

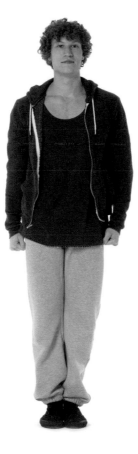

8

Jump, feet together, arms down, hands in fists, count 8

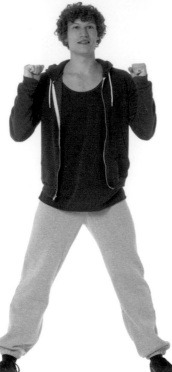

9

Step out with your left foot, fists in front of your shoulders, count 1

10

Bring your right foot to join the left, knees bent, and cross your arms, left over right, keeping them straight, in front of your chest, count 2

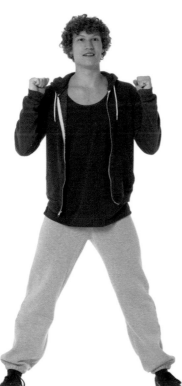

11

Step out with your right foot, fists in front of your shoulders, count 3

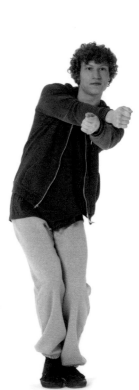

12

Bring your left foot to join the right, knees bent, and cross your arms, left over right, keeping them straight, in front of your chest, count 4

13

Step out with your left foot, fists in front of your shoulders, count 5

14

Bring your right foot to join the left, knees bent, and cross your arms, left over right, keeping them straight, in front of your chest, count 6

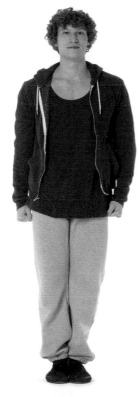

15

Jump, feet apart, and raise both arms, palms facing out, count 7

16

Jump, feet together, arms down, hands in fists, count 8

17

Step out with your right foot, right arm raised and palm facing up, left arm and palm facing down, keeping arms straight with flat hands, count 1

18

Step out with your left foot, left arm raised and palm facing up, right arm and palm facing down, keeping arms straight with flat hands, count 2

19

Step out with your right foot, right arm raised and palm facing up, left arm and palm facing down, keeping arms straight with flat hands, count 3

20

Bring your arms in, place your right hand on top of your left, keeping the palms flat, raise your right elbow, and relax your body, count 'and'

21

Step out with your right foot, right arm raised and palm facing up, left arm and palm facing down, keeping arms straight with flat hands, count 4

22

Step out with your left foot, left arm raised and palm facing up, right arm and palm facing down, keeping arms straight with flat hands, count 5

23

Step out with your right foot, right arm raised and palm facing up, left arm and palm facing down, keeping arms straight with flat hands, count 6

24

Step out with your left foot, left arm raised and palm facing up, right arm and palm facing down, keeping arms straight with flat hands, count 7

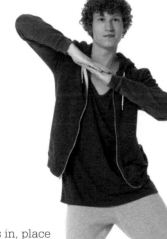

25

Bring your arms in, place your left hand on top of your right, keeping the palms flat, raise your left elbow, and relax your body, count 'and'

26

Step out with your left foot, left arm raised and palm facing up, right arm and palm facing down, keeping arms straight with flat hands, count 8

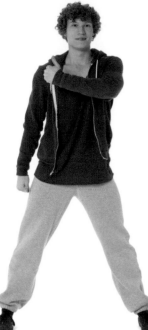

27

Step out with your right foot, right arm across your chest, a fist with thumb out in front of your left shoulder, left arm down, count 1

28

Bring your left foot in to join the right, knees bent, and move your right arm to the side and 'thumb' a lift, count 2

29

Step out with your left foot, left arm across your chest, a fist with thumb out in front of your right shoulder, right arm down, count 3

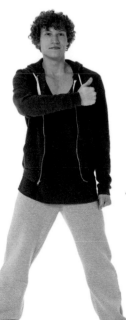

30

Bring your right foot in to join the left, knees bent, and move your left arm to the side and 'thumb' a lift, count 4

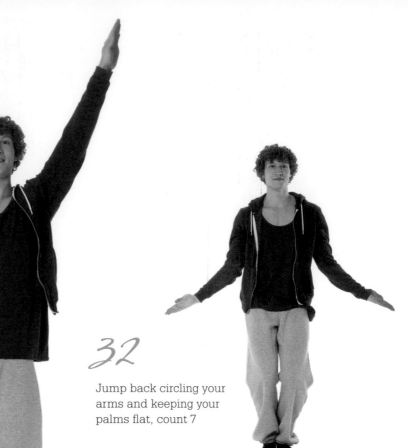

31

Jump forward with your arms raised, palms facing out, counts 5 hold 6

32

Jump back circling your arms and keeping your palms flat, count 7

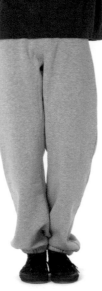

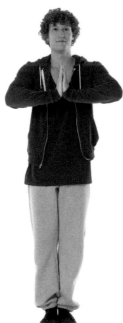

33

Close your hands together in 'prayer', legs straight, count 8.
Repeat steps 1–33

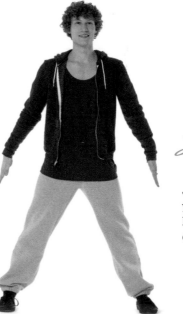

34

Jump, feet apart, keeping your arms low and your hands flat, palms facing in, count 1

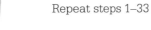

Go Go Go Joseph

35

Jump, feet together, and close your hands in 'prayer', count 2

36

Jump feet out, pointing forward, making a 'square' with your arms, and bending your legs, count 3

37

Jump, feet together, and close your hands in 'prayer', count 4

38

Jump feet out, leaning forward with your body and placing your hands on your legs, count 5

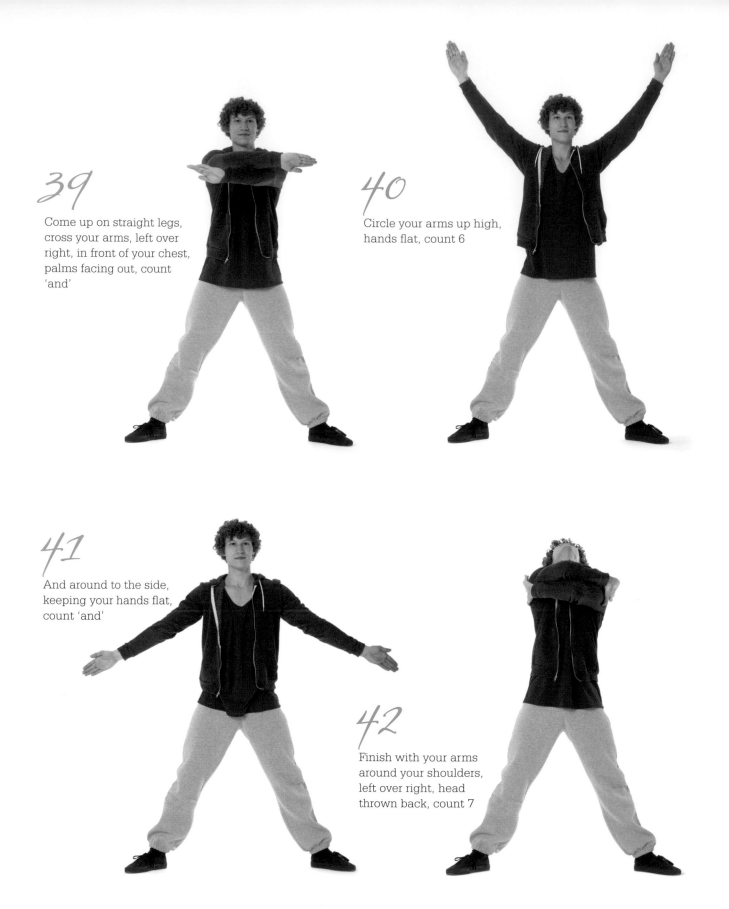

39

Come up on straight legs, cross your arms, left over right, in front of your chest, palms facing out, count 'and'

40

Circle your arms up high, hands flat, count 6

41

And around to the side, keeping your hands flat, count 'and'

42

Finish with your arms around your shoulders, left over right, head thrown back, count 7

43

Leaning forward with your
body and placing your hands
on your legs, count 8

44

Step to the right with
'square' arms, right palm
facing up, left facing
down, count 1

45

Step to the left with 'square' arms, left palm facing up, right facing down, count 2

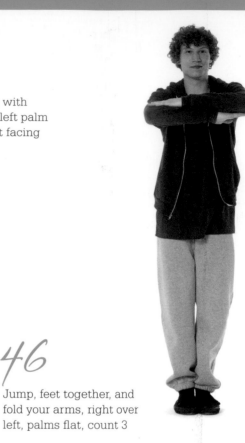

46

Jump, feet together, and fold your arms, right over left, palms flat, count 3

47

Step forward with your right foot and open your arms, keeping your elbows bent and palms facing down, count 4

48

Bend your knees, bring your arms back in and fold them, right over left, across your chest, count 5

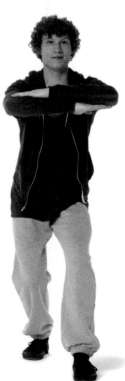

49

Turn your right leg out, lifting your toes off the floor, leaning your head and raising your right arm to the same side, count 6

50

Lower your foot, bring your right arm back in and straighten your body, count 7

51

Bring your right foot back to join the left, and lower your arms to your sides, palms facing forward, count 'and'

52

Circle your arms, finishing with your hands together in 'prayer' in front of your chest, count 8.
Repeat steps 34–52

As you build your stamina, repeat the entire routine from the beginning

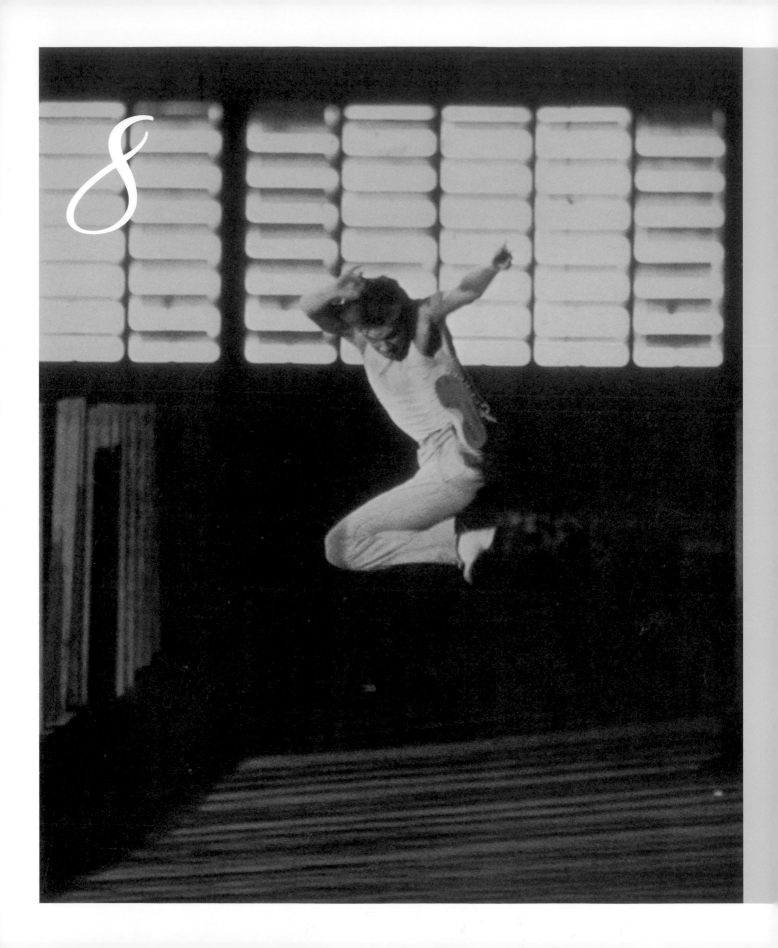

Footloose

Footloose

Written by Kenny Loggins

I saw the film as soon as it opened and watched Kevin Bacon burst on to the screen. He plays teenager Ren, who, with his mother, moves to Beaumont, a small town where dancing and rock 'n' roll has been banned, and he has to convince everyone why they should dance. What I remember most was the opening shot, where you see lots of different dancing feet doing every style of dance moving to the title track.

For me, dancing has never been about being famous. For as long as I can remember, I have just wanted to dance. I started with ballet, then later ballroom, tap and what used to be called 'modern dance'. All I could think about was getting to class. Dancing was my idea of heaven and I literally had to dance to live. With that in my DNA I could really empathise with the *Footloose* story line. If I had my way everyone in every town would be dancing! I often watch people walking on the street listening to music and automatically they are walking in time. Basically, walking is only one step away from dancing. With the new film adaptation of *Footloose* I can guarantee that legions of new young fans are going to be Footloose and fancy free. I heard a rumour that Madonna auditioned for the film! If it's true, I'd have loved to have been a fly on the wall!

> The fast fancy footwork will keep your brain thinking while your feet are constantly moving

The music for *Footloose* has a Country and Western feel to it, and some of the steps are from line dancing, as are the steps in my routine. The fast fancy footwork will keep your brain thinking while your feet are constantly moving. Once you have mastered the routine, you can keep repeating it to get a good work out – especially on tightening the thighs.

This line dance style routine will make you 'feel the burn' in your thighs, and your bottom will also feel the benefits. Find yourself a cowboy hat and have fun!

Stand with your weight on your right foot, hands on hips, ready to transfer your weight forward onto your left foot

1

Put your right heel out to the side, bend your left leg, and place your hands on your hips, count 1

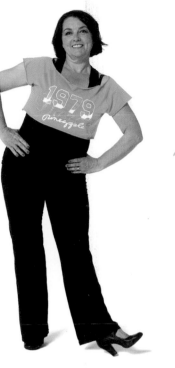

2

Bring your feet together, and straighten your legs, keeping your hands on your hips, count 2. Repeat steps 1 and 2, counts 3, 4

3

Still keeping your hands on your hips, put your left heel out to side, and bend your right leg, count 5

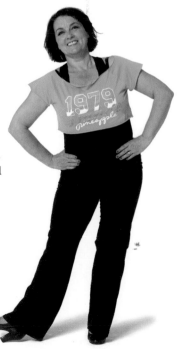

4

Bring your feet together, and straighten your legs, continuing to keep your hands on your hips, count 6. Repeat steps 3 and 4, counts 7, 8

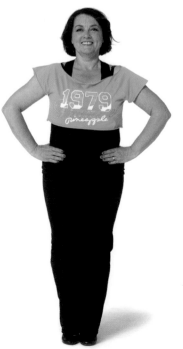

5

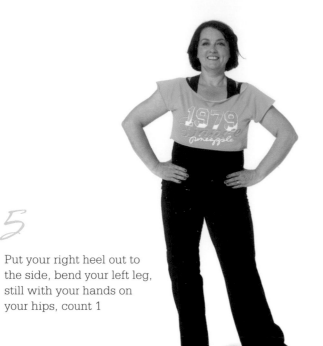

Put your right heel out to the side, bend your left leg, still with your hands on your hips, count 1

6

Switch onto the ball of your foot, count 2

7

Then back onto your heel, all the time continuing to keep your hands on your hips, count 3

8

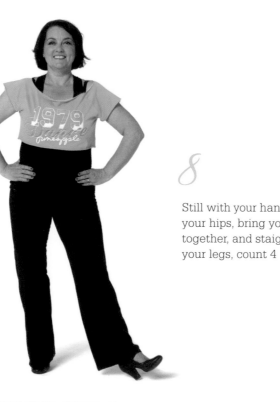

Still with your hands on your hips, bring your feet together, and staighten your legs, count 4

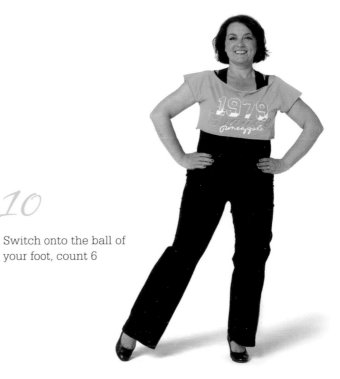

9

Put your left heel out to the side, and bend your right leg, hands still on hips, count 5

10

Switch onto the ball of your foot, count 6

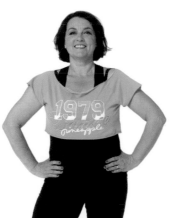

11

Switch back onto your heel, continuing to keep your hands on your hips, count 7

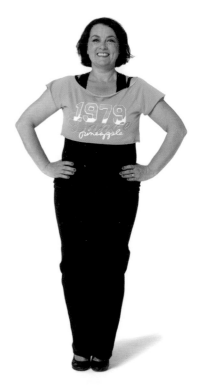

12

Bring your feet together again, count 8.
Repeat steps 1–12

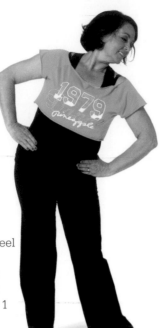

13

Step to the side on the heel of your right foot, bend your left knee, and, with hands still on hips, look down to the right, count 1

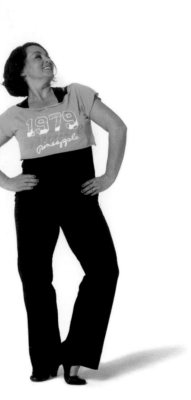

14

Bring your left foot next to your right, and transfer your weight onto it, right heel off the floor, and both knees bent, look up to the right, count 2

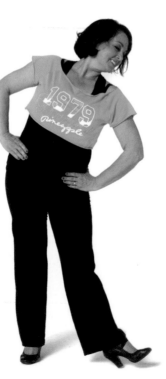

15

Step to the side on the heel of your right foot, bend your left knee, and, with hands on hips, look down to the right, count 3

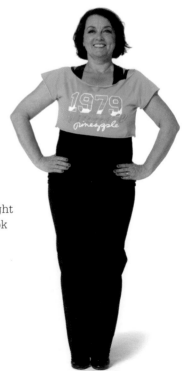

16

Bring your left foot together with your right foot, legs straight, look forward, count 4

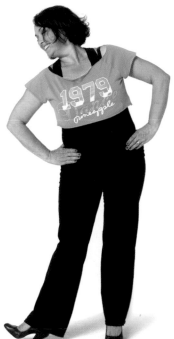

17

Step to the side on the heel of your left foot, bend your right knee, and, with hands on hips, look down to the left, count 5

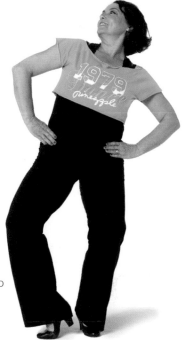

18

Bring your right foot next to your left, and transfer your weight onto it, left heel off the floor, both knees bent, and look up to the left, count 6

19

Step to the side on the heel of your left foot, bend your right knee, and, with hands on hips, look down to the left, count 7

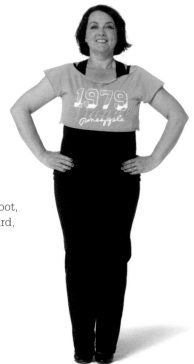

20

Bring your right foot together with your left foot, legs straight, look forward, count 8

21

Lift your right leg backward, and bend your left knee, at the same time touching the outside of your right foot with your right hand, and raising your left arm, count 1

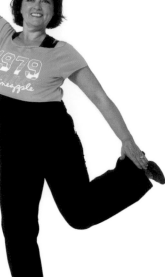

22

Twist your right leg forward, at the same time touching the inside of your right foot with your left hand, and raising your right arm, count 2

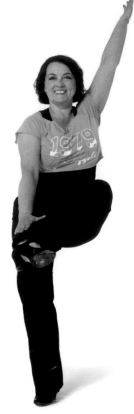

23

Twist your right leg backward, touch the outside of your right foot with your right hand, and raise your left arm, count 3

24

Bring your right leg down, so your feet are together, put your hands on your hips, and straighten your legs, count 4

25

Lift your left leg, backward bend your right knee, touch the outside of your left foot with your left hand, and raise your right arm, count 5

26

Twist your left leg forward, touch the inside of your left foot with your right hand, and raise your left arm, count 6

27

Twist your left leg backward, touch the outside of your left foot with your left hand, and raise your right arm, count 7

28

Bring your feet together, put your hands on your hips, and straighten your legs, count 8

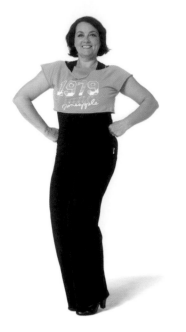

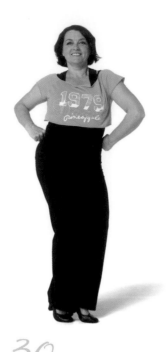

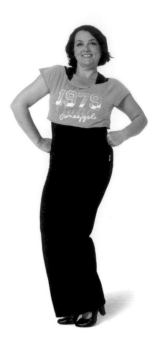

29

With your feet together, bend both knees, and push both your heels and hips to the right, fists on hips, count 1

30

Move your heels to the left side, almost stretch your knees, count 'and'

31

With your feet together, bend both knees, and push both your heels and hips to the right, fists on hips, count 2

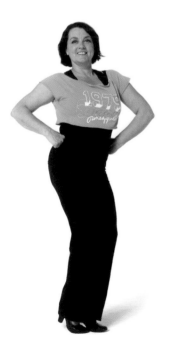

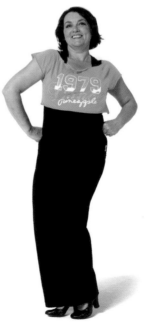

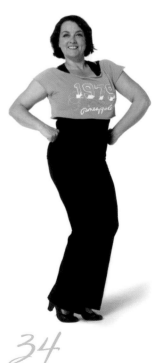

32

Bend both knees, and push both your heels and hips to the left, fists on hips, count 3

33

Move your heels to the right, almost stretch your knees, count 'and'

34

Bend both knees, and push both your heels and hips to the left, count 4

35

Push both your heels and hips to the right, further bending your knees, count 5

36

Push both your heels and hips to the left, bending knees even more, count 6

38

Come up to straight legs, keeping your feet together, count 8

37

Push once more to the right, getting even lower to the ground, count 7

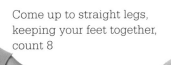

39

Push both your heels and hips to the left, and bend your knees, count 1

40

Push your heels and hips to the right, almost stretch your knees, count 'and'

41

Push both your heels and hips to the left, bend your knees, count 2

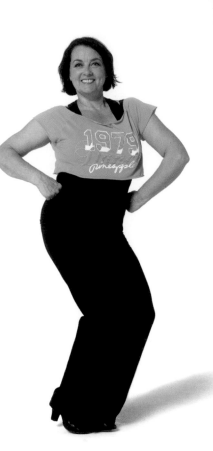

43

Move your heels and hips to the left, almost stretch your knees, count 'and'

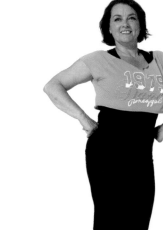

42

Push your heels and hips to the right, and bend your knees, count 3

44

Push your heels and hips to the right, bend your knees, count 4

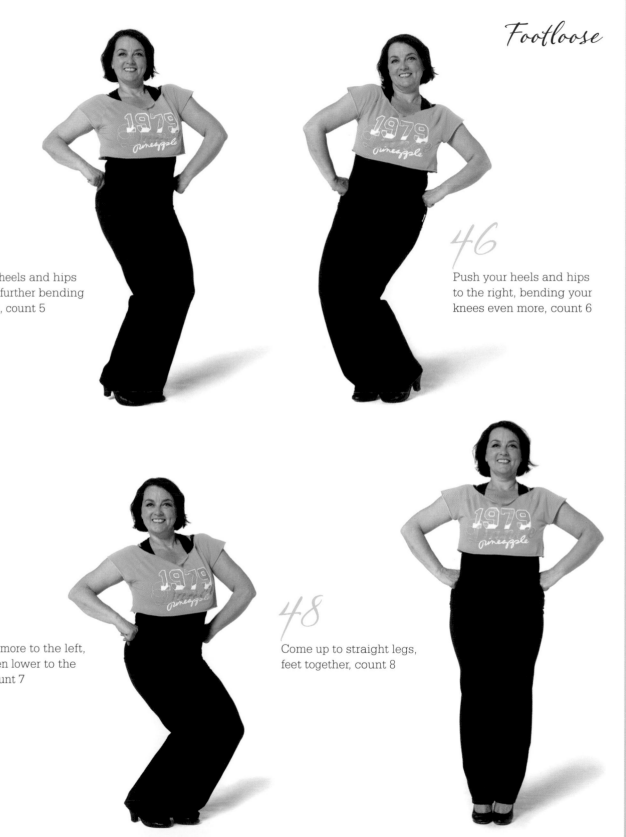

45

Push your heels and hips to the left, further bending your knees, count 5

46

Push your heels and hips to the right, bending your knees even more, count 6

47

Push once more to the left, getting even lower to the ground, count 7

48

Come up to straight legs, feet together, count 8

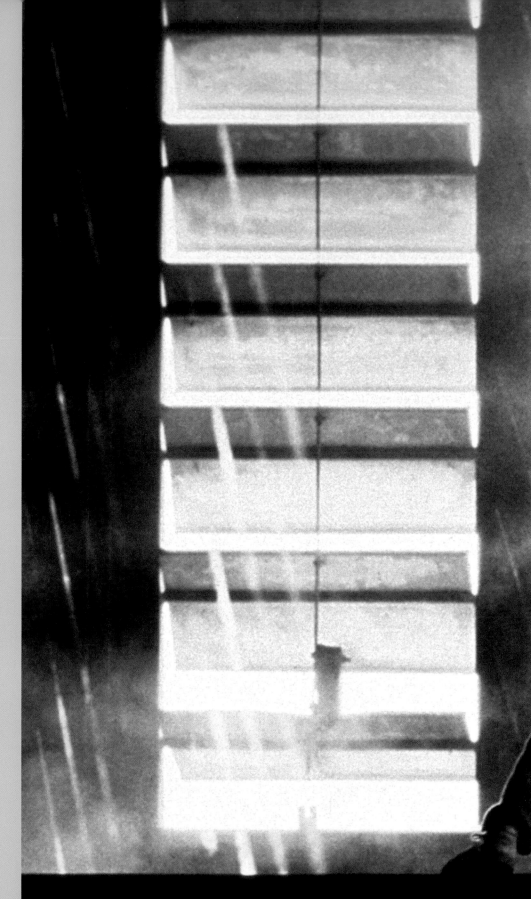

In a town where dancing is banned, Kevin Bacon cuts loose as he releases his frustrations through dance

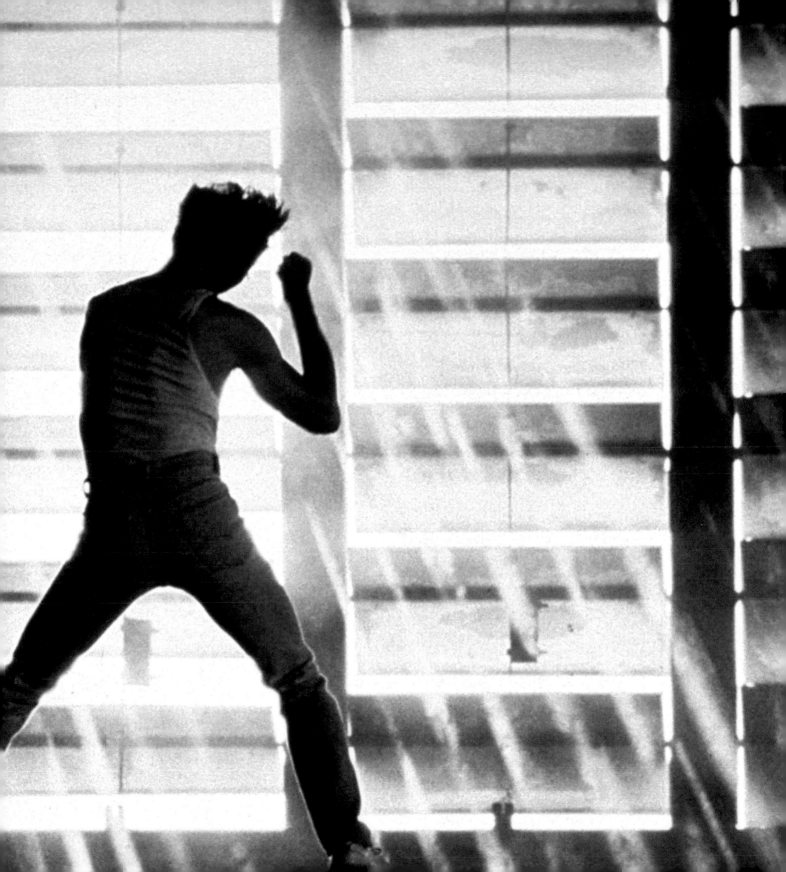

49

Step out onto the right heel, left leg bent, right leg straight, and, with hands on hips, look down to the right, count 1

50

Step onto your left foot, crossing behind the right foot, right heel off the floor, and look up to the right, count 2. Repeat steps 49 and 50, counts 3, 4

51

Jump onto your right foot, lift your left leg in the air to the side, and look to the front, count 5

52

Jump onto your left leg, lift your right leg in the air to the side, and look to the front, count 6

53

Hop on your left leg,
twisting your right leg
forward and out, count 7

54

Jump, landing with feet
together, hands on hips,
count 8

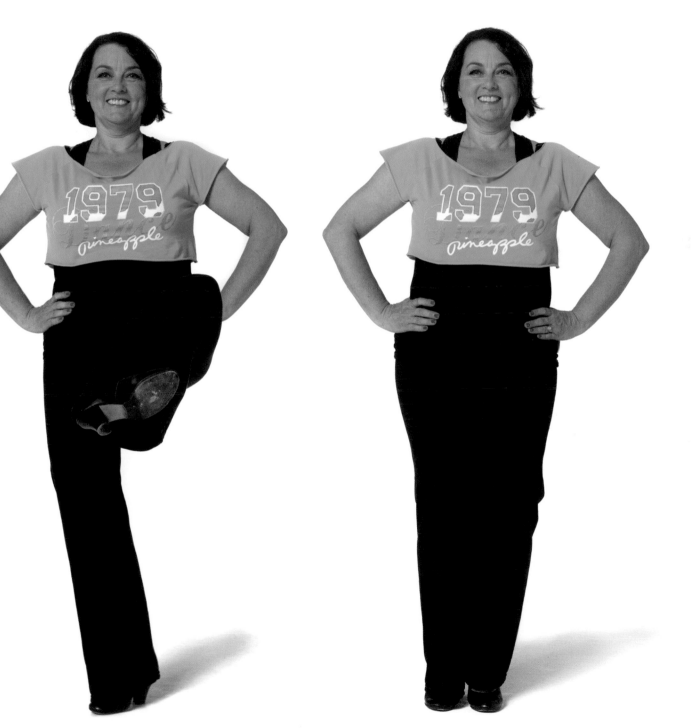

55

Step out onto your left heel, right leg bent, left leg straight, hands on hips, and look down to the left, count 1

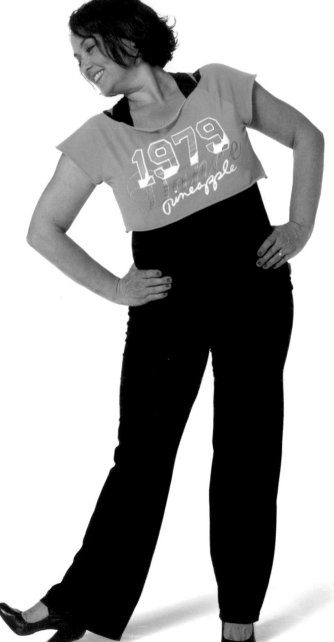

56

Step onto your right foot, crossing behind the left foot, left heel off the floor, and look up to the left, count 2. Repeat steps 55 and 56, counts 3, 4

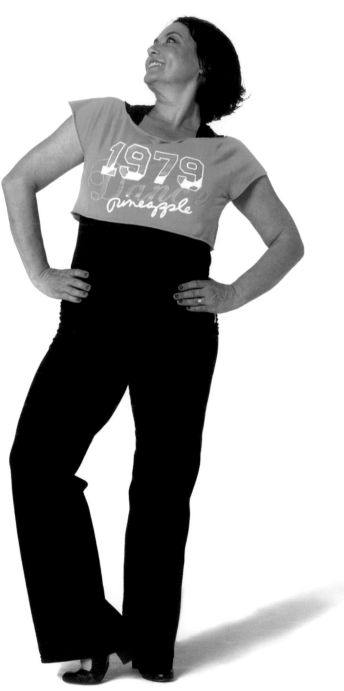

57

Jump onto your left foot, lift your right leg in the air to the side, and look to the front, count 5

58

Jump onto your right leg, lift your left leg in the air to the side, and look to the front, count 6

59

Hop on your right leg, twisting your left leg forward and out, count 7

60

Jump, landing with feet together, hands on hips, count 8. Repeat steps 49–60

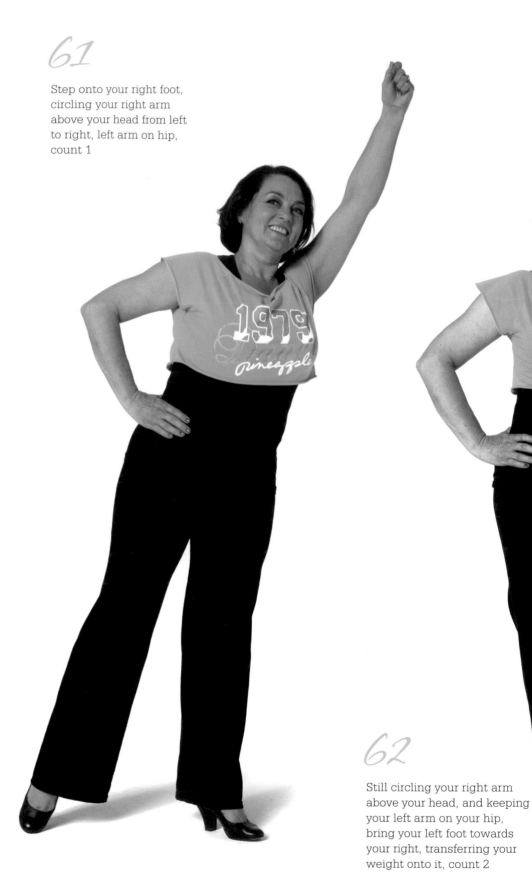

61

Step onto your right foot, circling your right arm above your head from left to right, left arm on hip, count 1

62

Still circling your right arm above your head, and keeping your left arm on your hip, bring your left foot towards your right, transferring your weight onto it, count 2

63

Still circling your right arm above your head, step onto your right leg, and lift your left foot off the floor, counts 3, 4

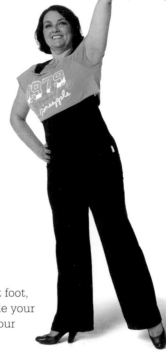

64

Step onto your left foot, continuing to circle your right arm above your head, count 5

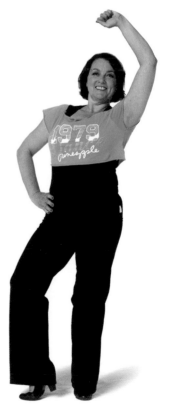

65

Bring your right foot towards your left, transferring weight onto it, continuing to circle your right arm above your head, count 6

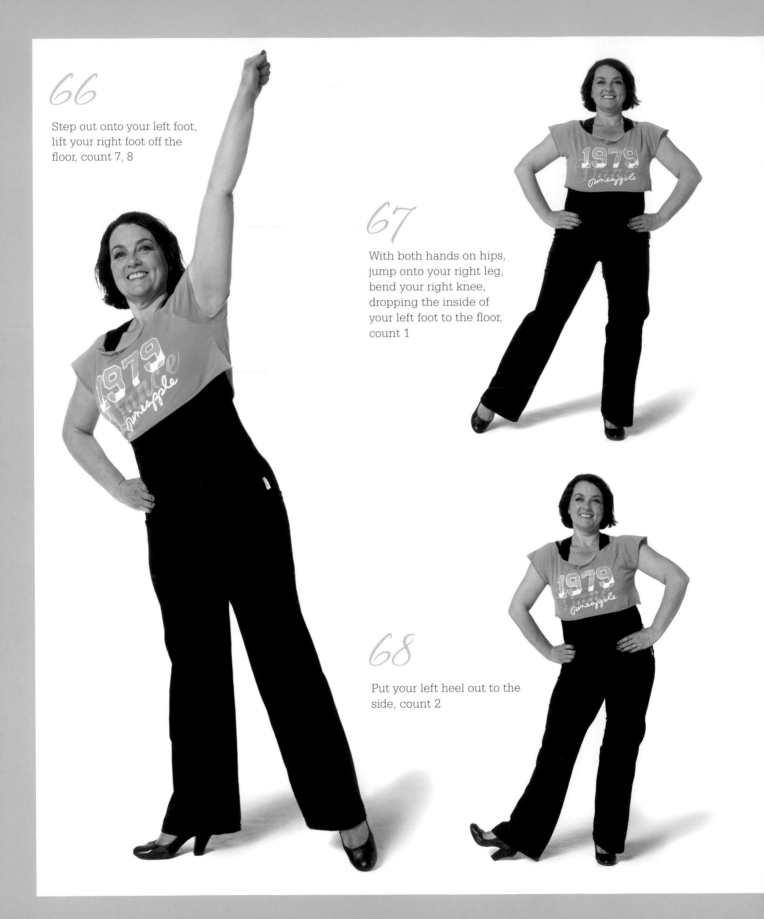

66

Step out onto your left foot, lift your right foot off the floor, count 7, 8

67

With both hands on hips, jump onto your right leg, bend your right knee, dropping the inside of your left foot to the floor, count 1

68

Put your left heel out to the side, count 2

69

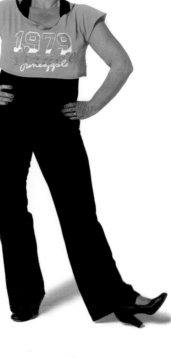

Still with both hands on hips, jump onto your left leg, and bend your left knee, dropping the inside of your right foot to the floor, count 3

70

Put your right heel out to the side, count 4.
Repeat steps 67 and 68, counts 5, 6

71

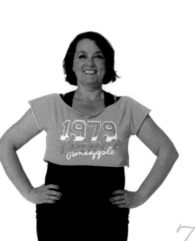

Jump feet together, bend knees, count 7

72

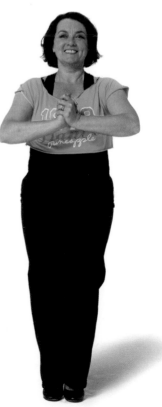

Clap hands, count 8.
Repeat steps 61–71

As you build your stamina, repeat the entire routine from the beginning

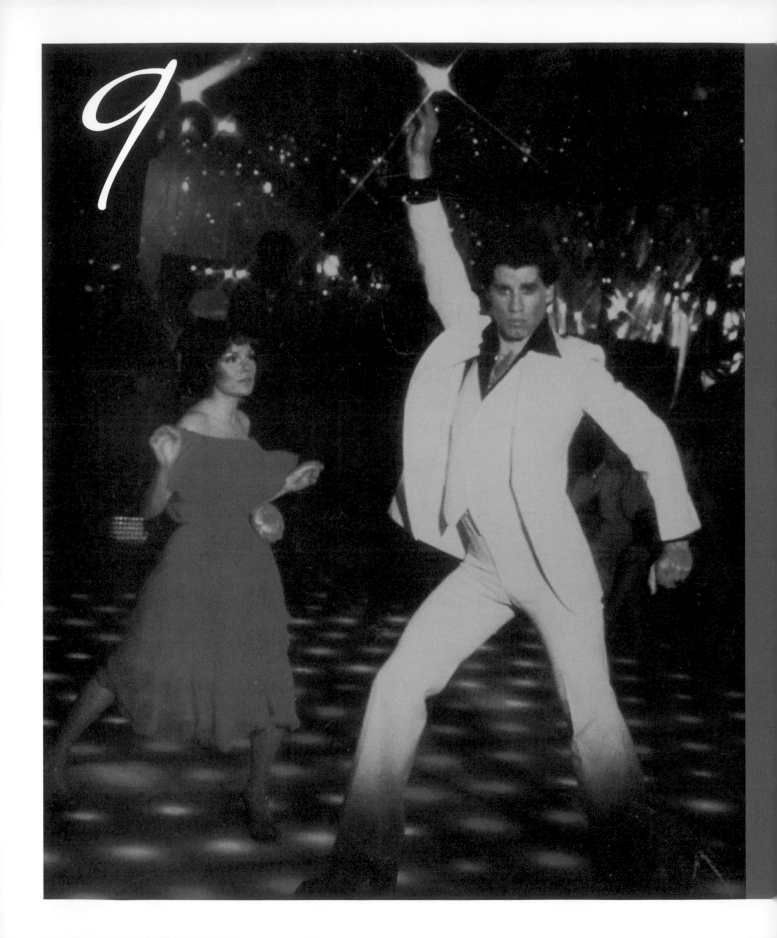

Saturday Night Fever

Night Fever

Written by Barry Gibb, Robin Gibb and Maurice Gibb

I always liken my own path to that of the lead character in *Saturday Night Fever*, Tony Manero. Tony thought that crossing the bridge from Brooklyn to Manhattan was a life journey. People from Brooklyn just didn't move to Manhattan. When I grew up in Manchester London was the big golden city. Just like Tony Manero, people I knew didn't go to London. I totally empathised with what it meant to cross the Brooklyn Bridge. Travelling by train or car from Manchester to London felt like travelling to another world.

The genius of John Travolta in the film was to make Tony – who was far from loveable – into a character with whom we all fall in love. Finding someone to play the role on stage was difficult. Our Tony had to dance, act *and* sing. The Bee Gees' songs from the film had to be sung live. Adam Garcia who had played Doody in *Grease* was Robert Stigwood's first choice. In fact I think Robert decided to stage *Saturday Night Fever* because he'd watched Adam in *Grease* and had seen something special. Doody isn't a big role, but when I took my nephew to see the show, he couldn't stop talking about Doody. Robert Stigwood was right, Adam was going to be a huge star, and he proved it on opening night at the London Palladium. When you're playing a small role in a musical and you're noticed as a stand out character it says a lot for your future career.

Everybody is familiar with John Travolta's moves to 'Night Fever', which are based on disco dance. It's a fun way to move – going from walking to dancing. The song also has a hypnotic beat which feels as natural as breathing. A good workout for arm, legs and also stomach muscles, my routine is a great one for face muscles too – picture John Travolta's famous pose and you can't help smiling.

> 'Night Fever' has a hypnotic beat that feels as natural as breathing. My routine is a good work out for your arms, legs and stomach muscles

Jump back into the 1970s with this fun disco dancing routine. A fantastic workout for your core muscles, this choreography requires good balance. Get the Fever!

Starting position: right leg to the side, put your weight on the ball of your foot, raise your right arm and point

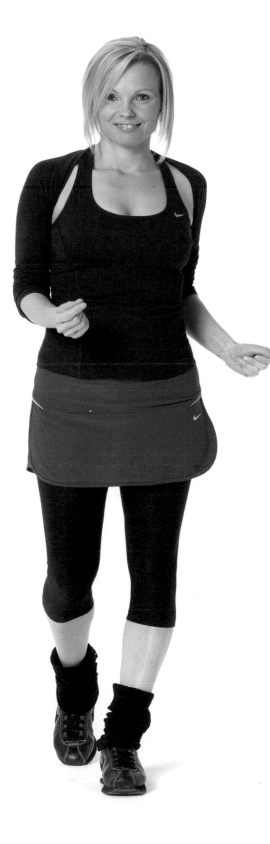

1

Walk forward with your
right foot, hands in fists,
elbows bent, count 1

Walk forward with your left foot, hands in fists, elbows bent, count 2

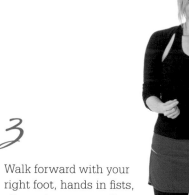

3

Walk forward with your right foot, hands in fists, elbows bent, count 3

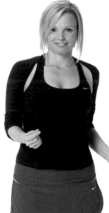

4

Touch your left foot to your right, knee bent, clap your hands in front of your chest, count 4

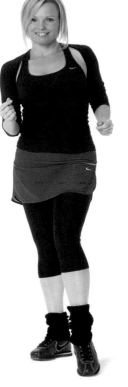

5

Step back on your left foot, arms by your sides, elbows bent, count 5

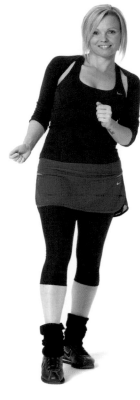

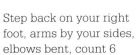

6

Step back on your right foot, arms by your sides, elbows bent, count 6

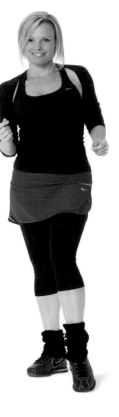

7

Step back on your left foot, arms by your sides, elbows bent, count 7

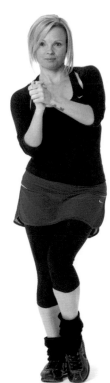

8

Touch your right foot to your left, knee bent, clap your hands in front of your chest, count 8

9

Step to the side with your right foot, left arm across your chest, right arm by your side, count 1

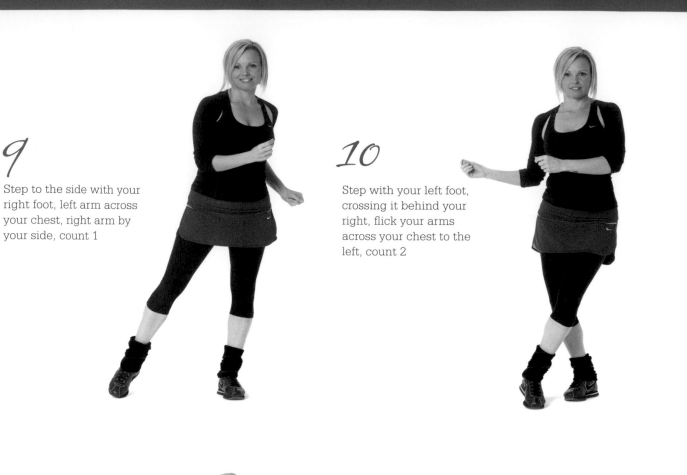

10

Step with your left foot, crossing it behind your right, flick your arms across your chest to the left, count 2

11

Step to the side with your right foot, left arm across your chest, right arm by your side, count 3

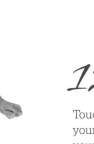

12

Touch your left foot to your right, knee bent, clap your hands in front of your chest, count 4

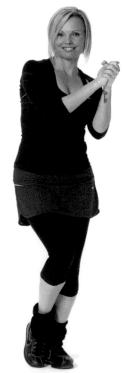

13

Step to the side with your left foot, right arm across your chest, left arm by your side, count 5

14

Step with your right foot, crossing it in front of your left, flick your arms across your chest to the right, count 6

15

Step to the side with your left foot, right arm across your chest, left arm by your side, count 7

16

Touch your right foot to your left, knee bent, clap your hands in front of your chest, count 8

17

Step onto your right foot, heel raised, look to the right, and bend your elbows so your arms are at right angles, count 1

18

Step onto your left foot, heel raised, look to the left, and bend your elbows so arms are at right angles, count 2

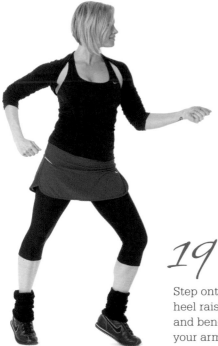

19

Step onto your right foot, heel raised, look to the right, and bend your elbows so your arms are at right angles, count 3

20

Drop onto your left foot, turn your face and your body to the front, and bend your left arm up, count 'and'

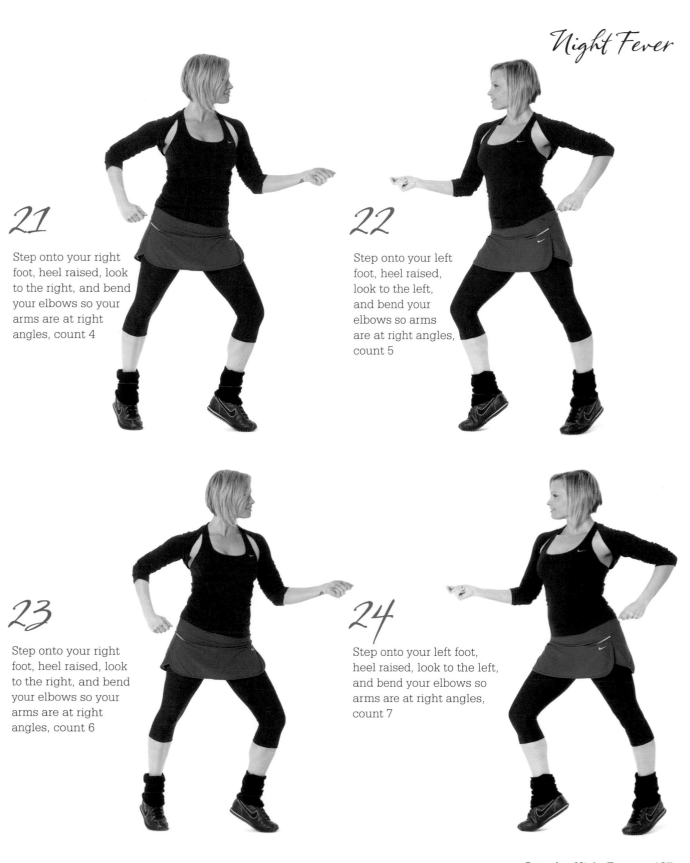

21

Step onto your right foot, heel raised, look to the right, and bend your elbows so your arms are at right angles, count 4

22

Step onto your left foot, heel raised, look to the left, and bend your elbows so arms are at right angles, count 5

23

Step onto your right foot, heel raised, look to the right, and bend your elbows so your arms are at right angles, count 6

24

Step onto your left foot, heel raised, look to the left, and bend your elbows so arms are at right angles, count 7

25

Drop onto your right foot, turn your face and your body to the front, and bend your right arm up, count 'and'

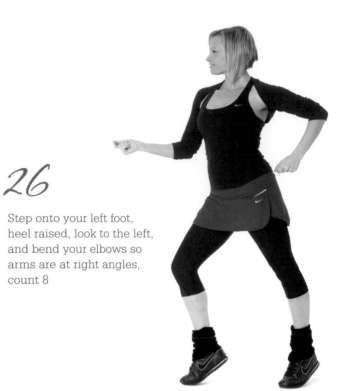

26

Step onto your left foot, heel raised, look to the left, and bend your elbows so arms are at right angles, count 8

27

Swivel to the left, bend your left knee, raise your left arm, finger pointed, and place your right hand on your hip, count 1

28

Swivel to the right, point your left arm down across your body, count 2

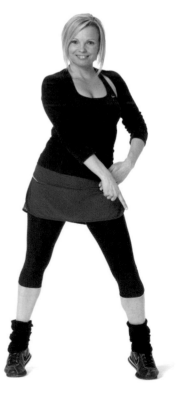

29

Swivel to the left, bend
your left knee, raise your
left arm, finger pointed,
your right hand still
on your hip, counts 3
hold 4

30

Swivel to the right, point
your left arm down across
your body, count 5

31

Swivel to the left, bend
your left knee, raise your
left arm, finger pointed,
your right hand still
on your hip, count 6

32

Swivel to the right, point
your left arm down across
your body, counts 7, hold 8.
Repeat steps 1–32

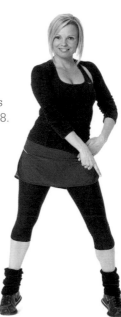

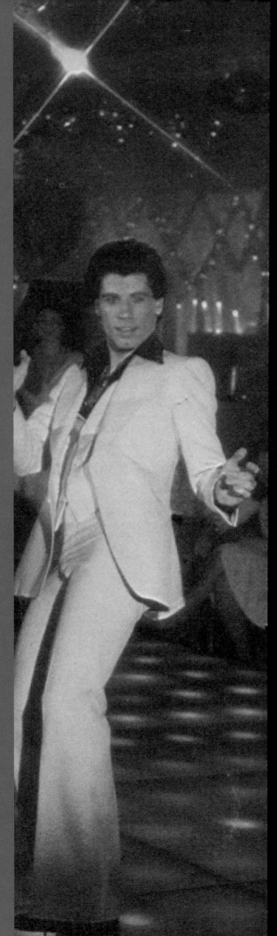
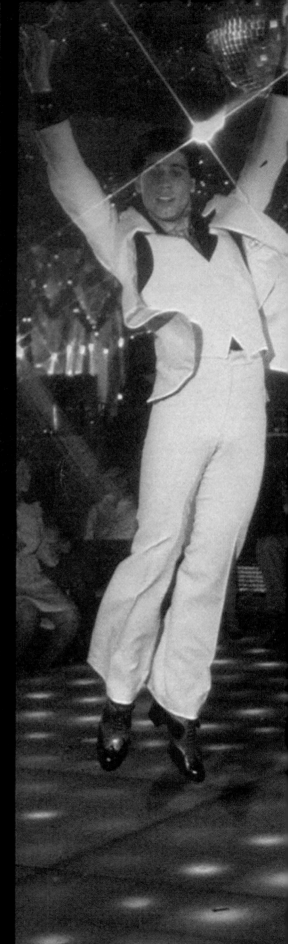

These images of John Travolta really make you want to move. He started a worldwide dance craze when he took to the disco floor in his white suit

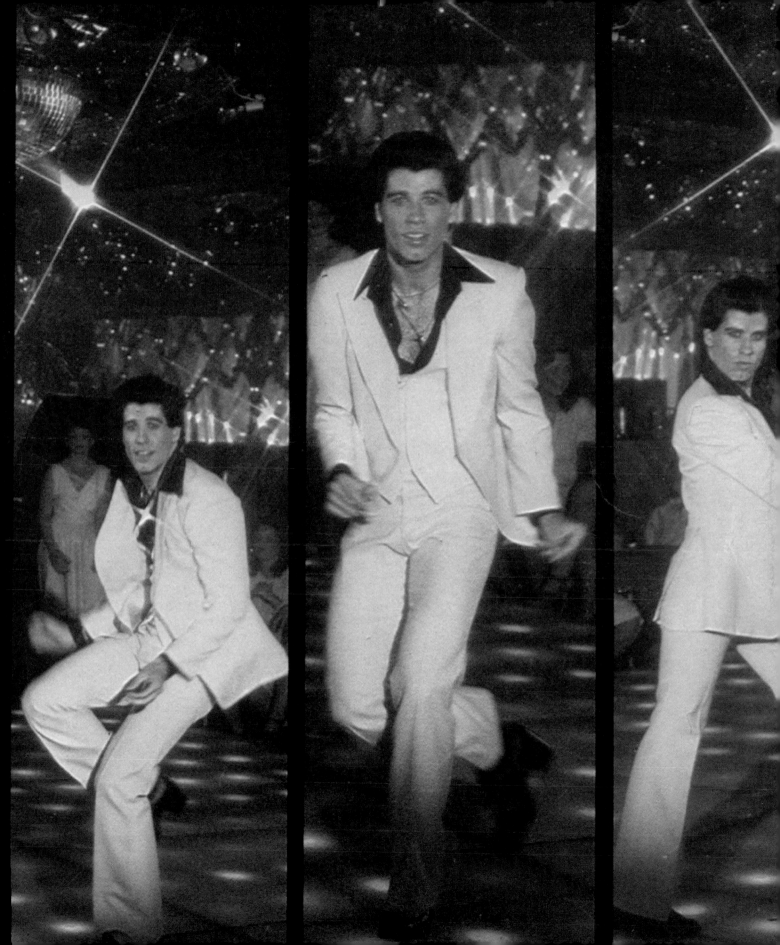

33

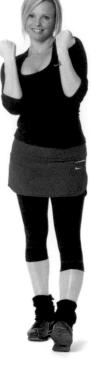

Put your left foot forward, heel on the floor, and raise both arms palms facing out, count 1

34

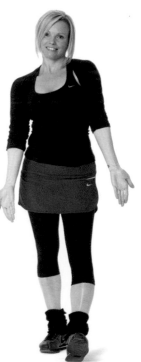

Switch and put your right foot forward, heel on the floor, and bring your arms into your chest, fists on your shoulders, count 2

35

Switch so your left foot is forward, and push your arms out to side, palms facing back, count 3

36

Switch so your right foot is forward, and bring your arms down to your sides, palms facing out, count 4. Repeat steps 33–37, counts 5, 6, 7, 8

37

Move your right leg out to the side, transfer your weight onto your left leg, raise both arms and click your fingers, count 1

38

Move your left leg out to the side, transfer your weight onto your right leg, raise both arms and click your fingers, count 2

39

Transfer your weight back onto your left foot, and lower your arms to the left, clicking your fingers, count 3

40

Bend both knees, count 'and'

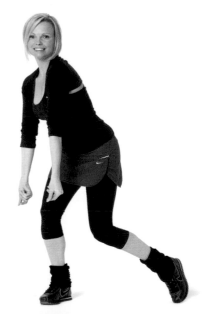

41
Stretch both legs, and click your fingers, count 4

42
Transfer your weight onto your right leg, raise both arms and click your fingers, count 5

43
Switch to the other side, transferring your weight onto your left leg, and click your fingers, count 6

44

Switch to the other side, transferring your weight onto your right leg, lower your arms, and click your fingers, count 7

45

Bend both knees and click your fingers, count 'and'

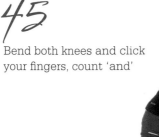

46

Stretch both legs, and click your fingers, count 8. Repeat steps 33–46

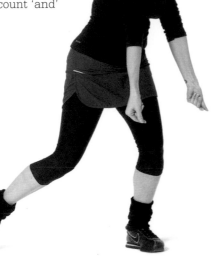

47

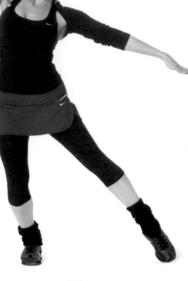

Transfer your weight onto your left leg, slide your right leg out, put your right arm out to the side, raise your left arm, and bend it so your hand is in front of your shoulder, palm facing down, count 1

48

Bring your right foot to join the left, clap hands in front of your chest, count 2

49

Put your weight onto your right leg, slide your left leg out, put your left arm out to the side, raise your right arm, and bend it so your hand is in front of your shoulder, palm facing down, count 3

50

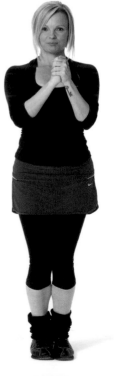

Bring your left foot to join the right, and clap your hands in front of your chest, count 4. Repeat steps 47–50, counts 5, 6, 7, 8

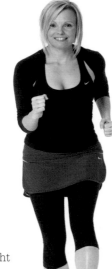
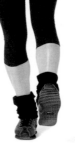

51

Kick your right foot forward with a straight leg, and bend your arms, left arm forward, right arm back, count 1

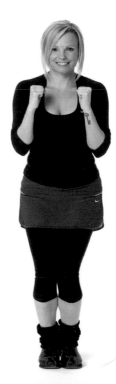

52

Bring your right foot back so your feet are joined together, and bend your arms into your chest so your fists are on your shoulders, count 'and'

53

Twist your legs, so your knees meet and your heels go out, and lift your elbows, keeping your arms bent, count 2

54

Twist your feet back together, bend your knees, and lower your elbows so your fists are on your shoulders, count 3

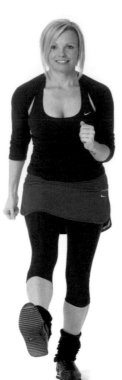

55

Kick your left foot forward
with a straight leg, and
bend your arms, right arm
forward, left arm back,
count 3

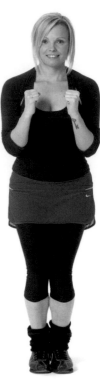

56

Bring your left foot back
so your feet are joined
together, and bend your
arms into your chest,
so your fists are on your
shoulders, count 'and'

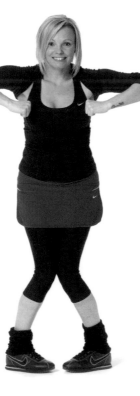

57

Twist your legs, so your
knees meet and your
heels go out, and lift your
elbows, keeping your arms
bent, count 4

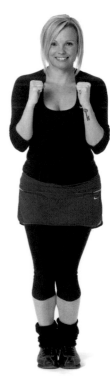

58

Twist your feet back
together, bend your knees,
and lower your elbows
so your fists are on your
shoulders, count 'and'

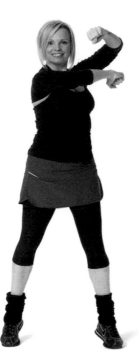

59

Step onto your right foot, with your left heel off the floor, body facing the right corner, and roll your arms, count 5

60

Bring your left foot to join your right, bend your knees, continuing to roll your arms, count 'and'. Repeat steps 59 and 60, counts 6 'and'

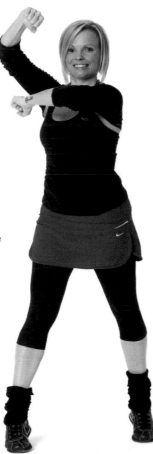

61

Step onto your left foot, with your right heel off the floor, body facing the left corner, continuing to roll your arms, count 7

62

Bring your right foot to join your left, bend your knees, continuing to roll your arms, count 'and'. Repeat steps 61 and 62, counts 8 and 'and'. Repeat steps 47–62

As you build your stamina, repeat the entire routine from the beginning

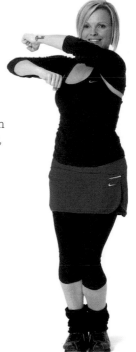

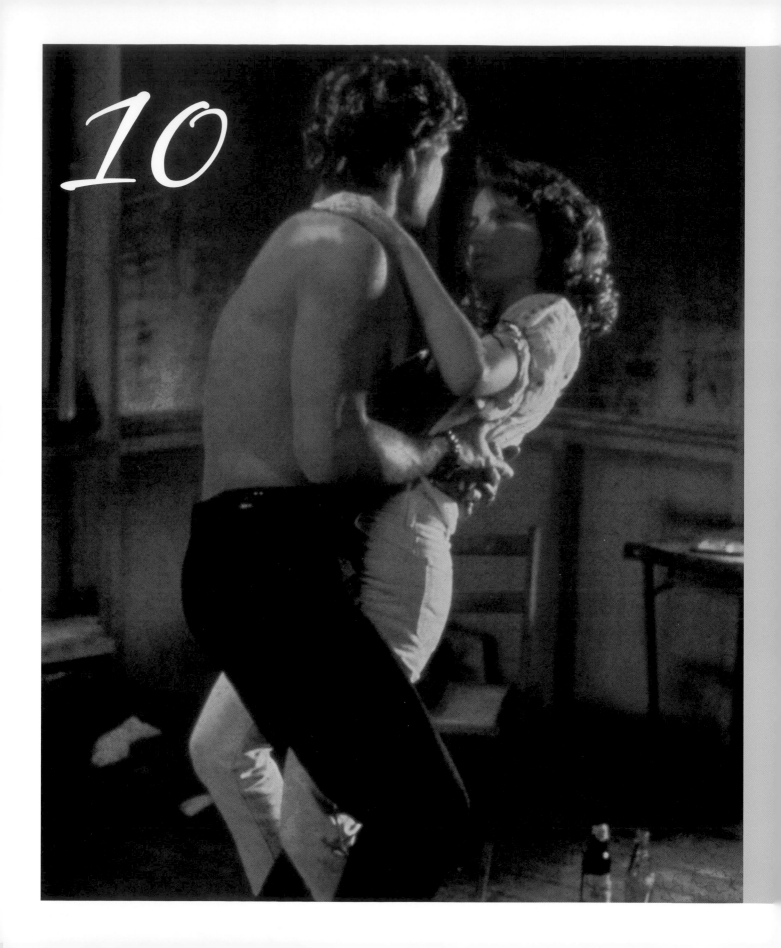

Dirty Dancing

The Time of My Life

Written by Franke Previte, John DeNicola and Donald Markowitz

The words Dirty Dancing say one thing to me – the late, great Patrick Swayze, who was responsible for hundreds of boys wanting to dance like him. He was every female dancer's dream – a gentleman who led his partner, making even the most flat-footed believe that they could dance. The choreography for the film was by Kenny Ortega, who I met in the late 70s when his group, The Tubes, were on tour in the UK. Kenny came as often as he could to see Hot Gossip and I was definitely a Tubes fan.

I've always thought Kenny's choreography for *Dirty Dancing* was some of the sexiest, most innovative ever seen in a movie. Who doesn't remember the moment Patrick Swayze jumps off the stage and, with those astonishingly seductive hip movements, sashays his way down the aisle? Kenny went on to do similarly ground-breaking work for Cher and was choreographing the legendary Michael Jackson Tour when the star died. Kenny went on to direct the memorial tribute in Los Angeles, which was broadcast to millions.

Patrick Swayze loved dance and exercise and was reputed to be up at 6am every morning to work out! Most of his dance movements ought to come with a label saying 'Don't try this at home!' My routine, however, is much simpler. It's based on mambo moves and, even though it's a cool-down, will make you feel really alive. Breathe in, pull up, breathe out, relax, to achieve the perfect posture and body line.

My routine for Dirty Dancing has a mambo feel and even though it's intended as a cool-down will make you feel really alive

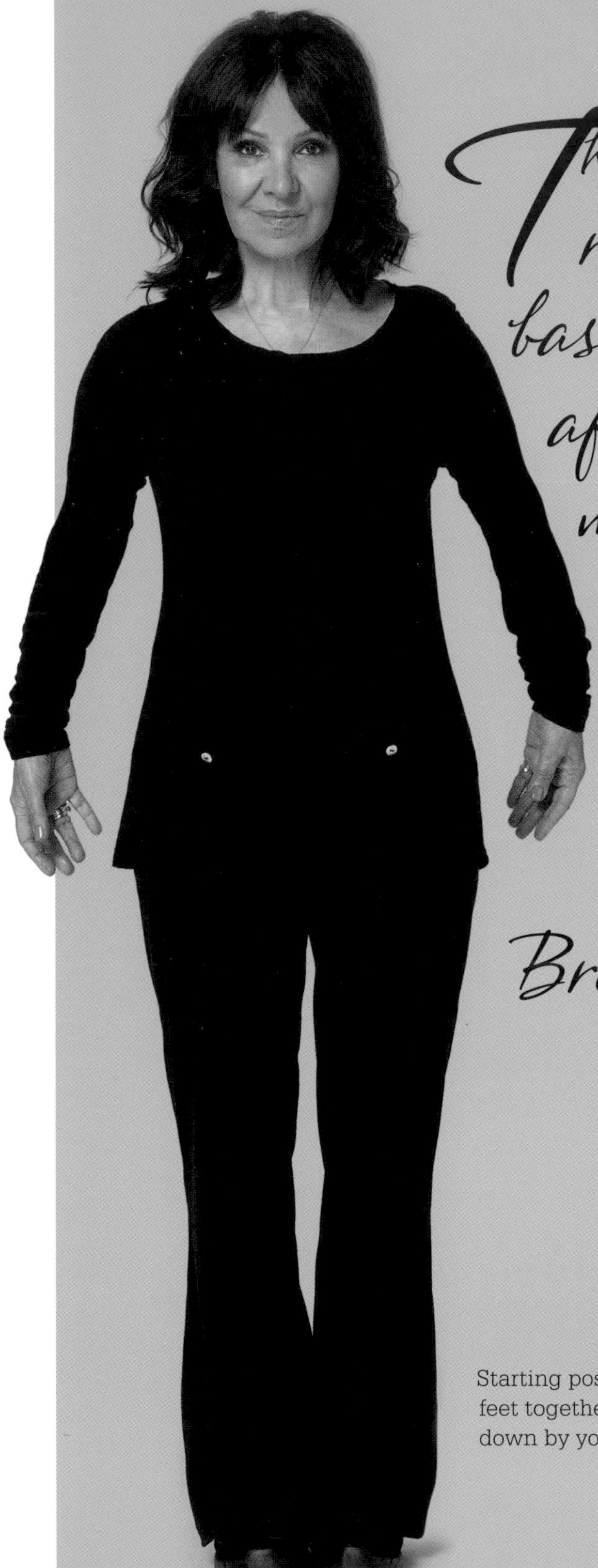

This is a gentle cool-down routine to help maintain basic breath control after a physical dance workout. It also gives a nice body stretch whilst at the same time allowing you to master your hot mambo steps. Breathe easy, stay cool.

Starting position:
feet together, arms
down by your sides

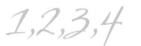

1,2,3,4

Open your right foot to the side. Bend your knees, legs apart. Take your arms in to your chest, then open them out to the side and up above your head, counts 1, 2, 3 , 4

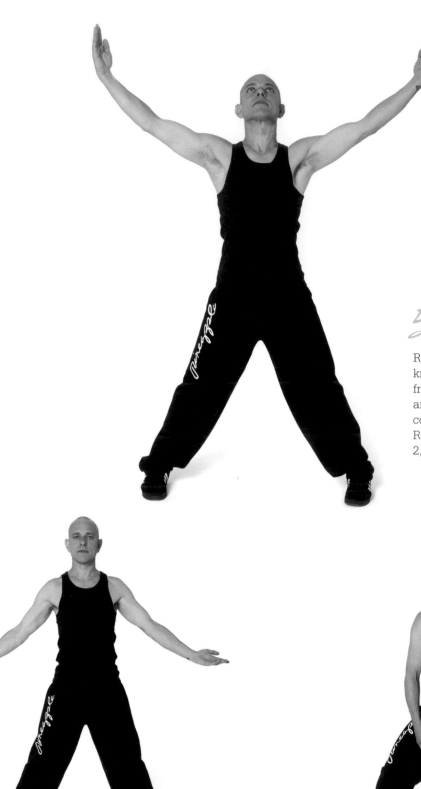

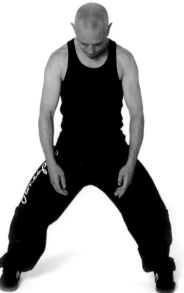

5,6,7

Relax and bend your
knees with your arms in
front. Take your arms out
and down to your sides,
counts 5, 6, 7, 8.
Repeat steps 1–7, counts 1,
2, 3, 4, 5, 6, 7, 8

8,9,10,11

Lift your right arm out to the side and stretch it up and over your head to the left, following your hand with your head and finish facing the front, counts 1, 2, 3, 4

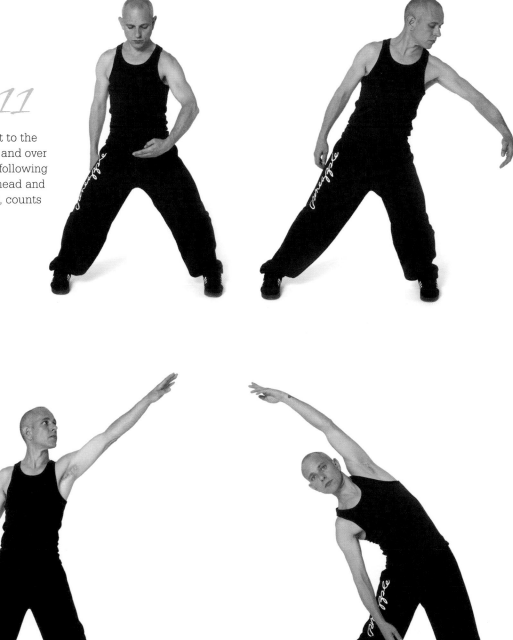

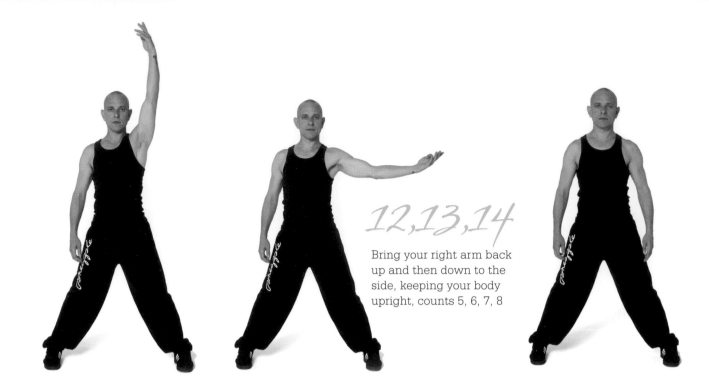

12,13,14

Bring your right arm back up and then down to the side, keeping your body upright, counts 5, 6, 7, 8

15,16,17,18

Bend your knees and lift your left arm to the side, stretching it up and over your head, following your hand with your head and finishing facing the front, counts 1, 2, 3, 4

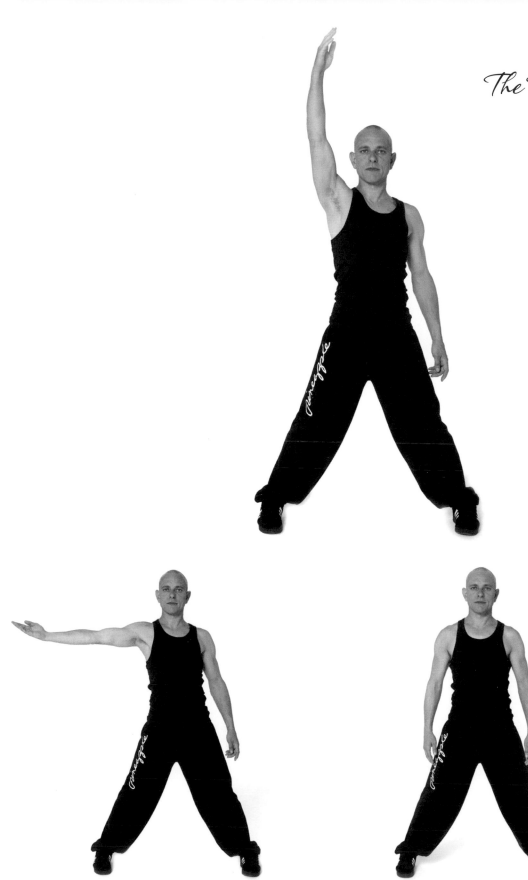

19,20,21

Raise your left arm and then bring it down to your side, keeping your body upright, counts 5, 6, 7, 8. Repeat steps 1–21

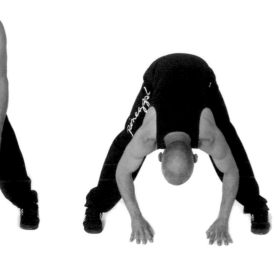

Starting with your head, gradually roll your body forwards until you are gently touching the floor with your fingers, counts 1, 2, 3, 4, 5, 6, 7, 8

25

Bend your knees, counts 1, 2, 3, 4

26

Stretch your knees, counts 5, 6, 7, 8.
Repeat steps 25 and 26, counts 1, 2, 3, 4, 5, 6, 7, 8

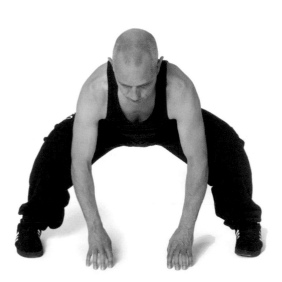

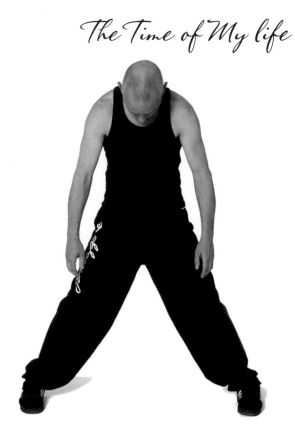

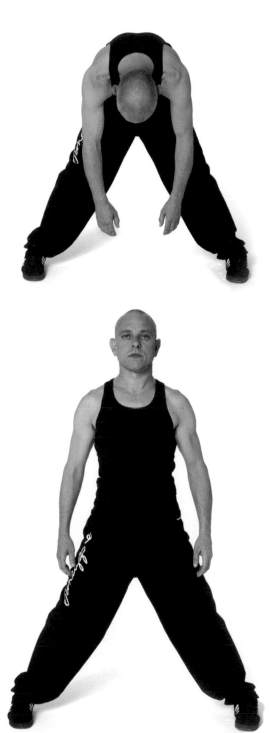

27, 28, 29

Slowly roll your body up,
finishing upright, arms by
your sides, counts 1, 2, 3,
4, 5, 6, 7, 8.
Repeat steps 22–29

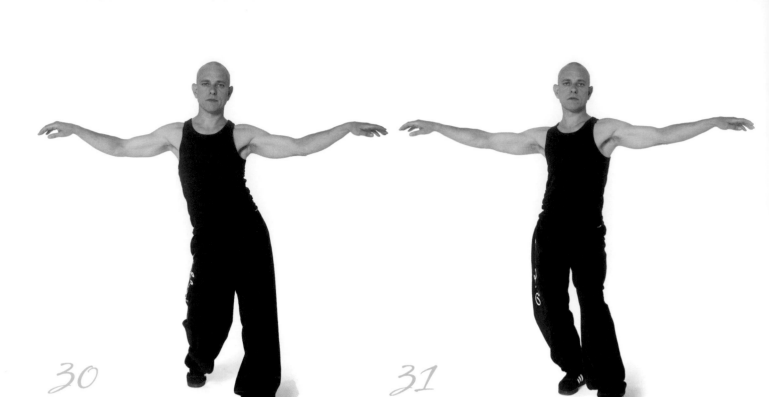

30

Step forward onto your right foot, right hip out, arms relaxed out to the sides at shoulder height, count 1

31

Transfer your weight onto your left foot, twisting your hips to the left, count 2

32

Bring your right foot back to join the left, count 3

33

Lift your heels off the floor, count 4

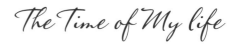

34 Step forward onto your left foot, left hip out, arms relaxed out to the sides, count 5

35 Transfer your weight onto your right foot, twisting your hips to the right, count 6

36 Bring your left foot back to join the right, count 7

37 Lift your heels off the floor, count 8. Repeat steps 30–37, counts 1, 2, 3, 4, 5, 6, 7, 8

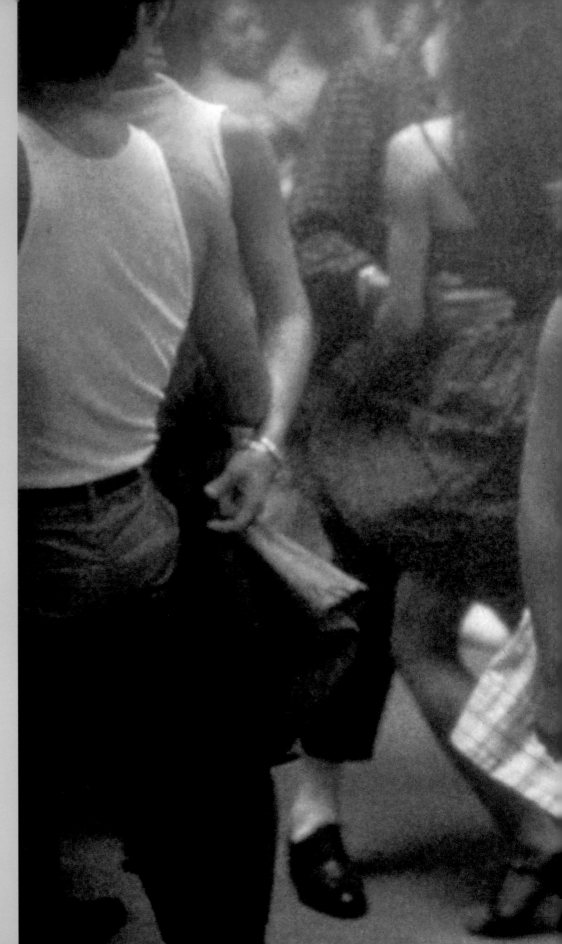

In this image from the film, you can feel movement and the heat from Patrick Swayze's hips. It truly was Dirty Dancing

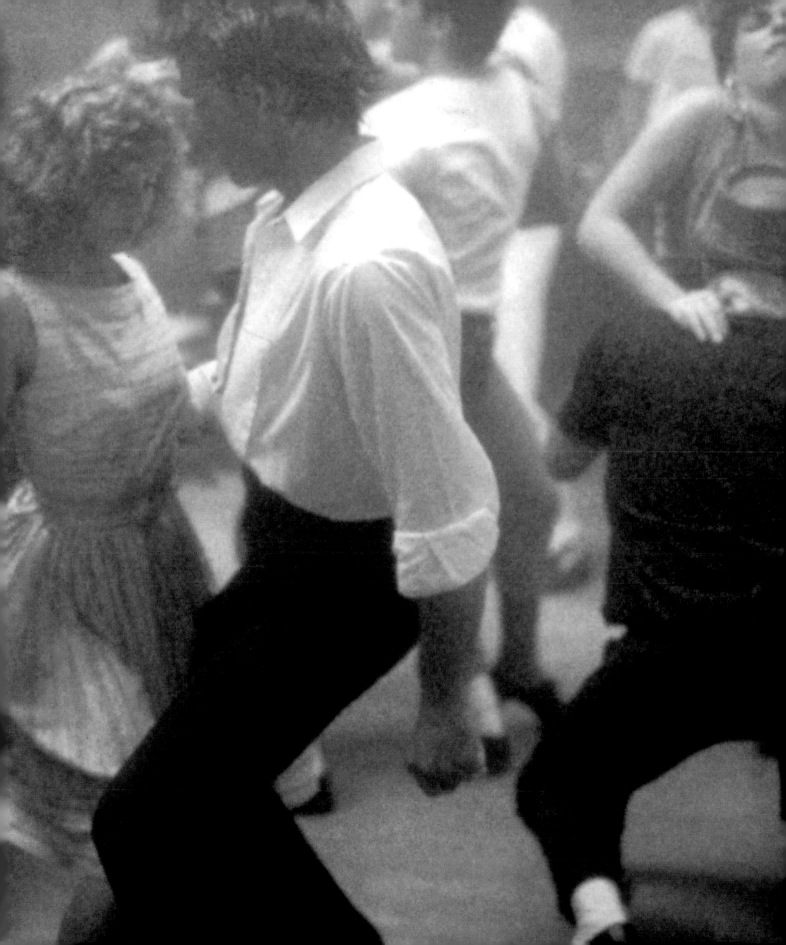

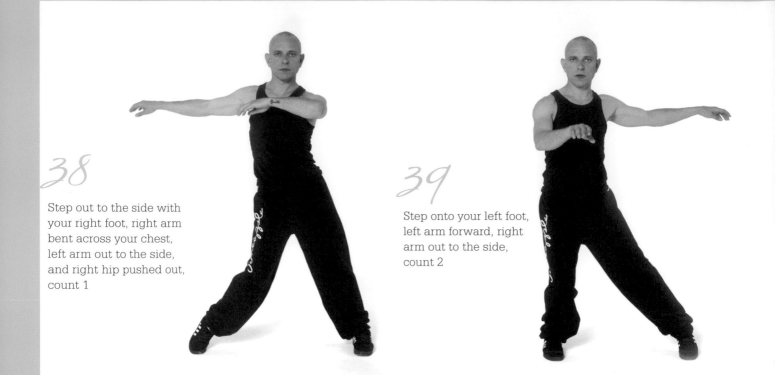

38

Step out to the side with your right foot, right arm bent across your chest, left arm out to the side, and right hip pushed out, count 1

39

Step onto your left foot, left arm forward, right arm out to the side, count 2

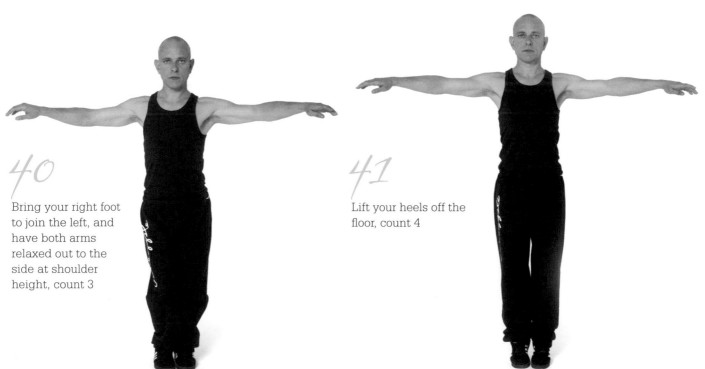

40

Bring your right foot to join the left, and have both arms relaxed out to the side at shoulder height, count 3

41

Lift your heels off the floor, count 4

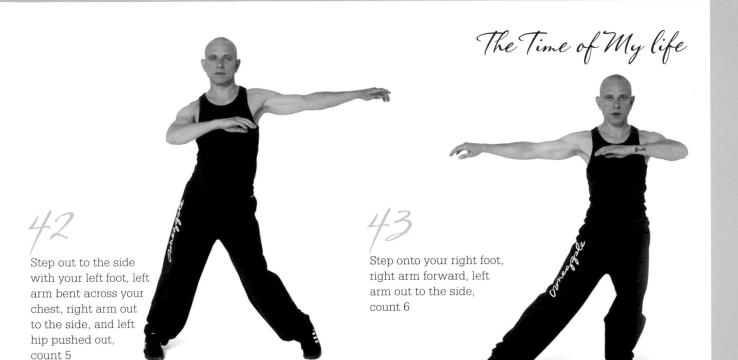

42

Step out to the side with your left foot, left arm bent across your chest, right arm out to the side, and left hip pushed out, count 5

43

Step onto your right foot, right arm forward, left arm out to the side, count 6

44

Bring your left foot to join the right, and have both arms relaxed out to the side, count 7

45

Lift your heels off the floor, count 8. Repeat steps 38–45, counts 1, 2, 3, 4, 5, 6, 7, 8

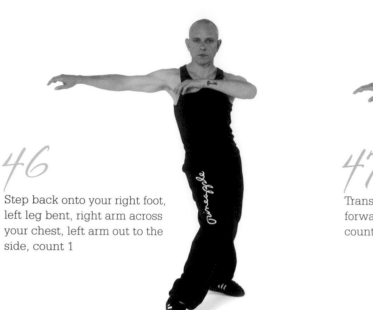

46

Step back onto your right foot,
left leg bent, right arm across
your chest, left arm out to the
side, count 1

47

Transfer your weight
forward onto your left foot,
count 2

48

Bring your right foot
forward to join the left,
knees bent, count 3

49

Lift your heels off the
floor, count 4

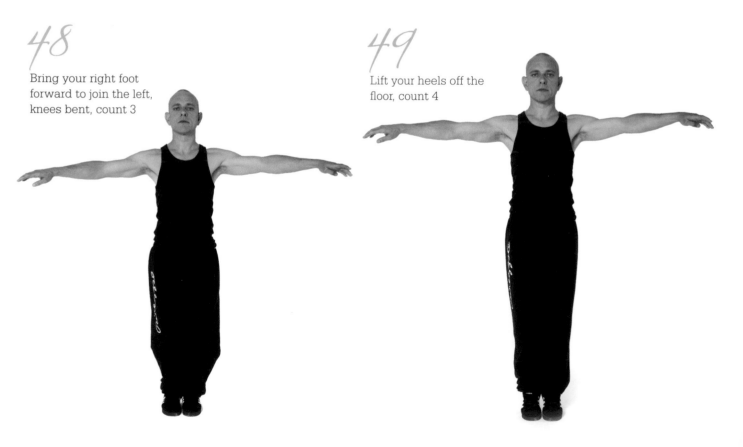

50

Step back with your left foot, left arm forward across your chest, count 5

51

Transfer your weight forward onto your right foot, both arms out to the side, count 6

52

Bring your left foot forward to join your right, count 7

53

Lift your heels off the floor, count 8.
Repeat steps 46–53, counts 1, 2, 3, 4, 5, 6, 7, 8.
Repeat steps 38–45, counts 1, 2, 3, 4, 5, 6, 7, 8

Step forward onto your
right foot, right hip out,
arms relaxed out to
the sides at shoulder
height, counts 1, 2

Step back with your right
foot, right arm forward
across your chest,
counts 3, 4

Step out to the side with
your right foot, counts 5, 6

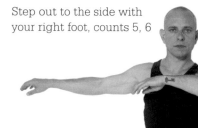

Bring your right foot to join
the left, rise up on your
toes, heels off floor,
counts 7, 8

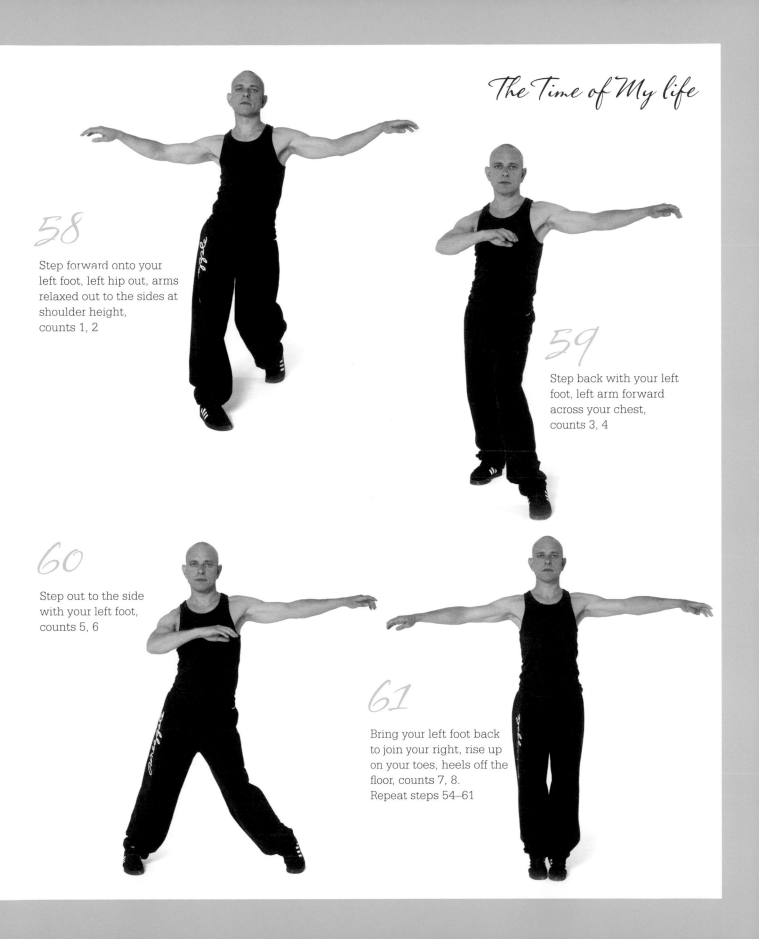

58

Step forward onto your left foot, left hip out, arms relaxed out to the sides at shoulder height, counts 1, 2

59

Step back with your left foot, left arm forward across your chest, counts 3, 4

60

Step out to the side with your left foot, counts 5, 6

61

Bring your left foot back to join your right, rise up on your toes, heels off the floor, counts 7, 8. Repeat steps 54–61

62

Step out to the side with your right foot, both arms above your head, and circle your arms forward and to the right, count 1

63

Bring your left foot to join the right, circling your arms back and to the left, count 2.
Repeat steps 62 and 63, counts 3, 4

64

Step out with your right foot, circle your arms above your head and to the right, count 5

65

Continue to circle your arms back and to the left, keeping your feet in the same position, count 6

66

Bring your left foot to join your right, circle your arms to the right, also looking to the right, counts 7, hold 8

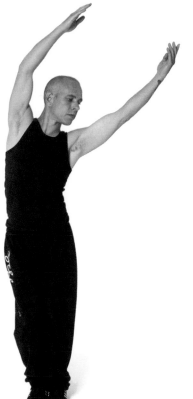

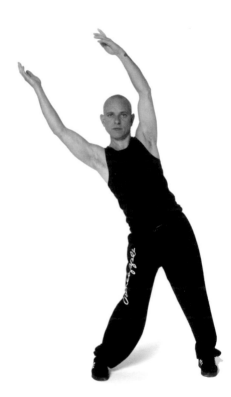

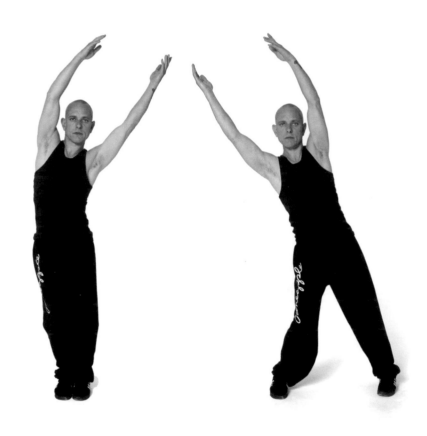

67

Step out to the side with your left foot, circling your arms to the left, count 1

68

Bring your right foot to join the left, and circle your arms to the right, count 2. Repeat steps 67 and 68, counts 3, 4

69

Step out with your left foot, and circle your arms to the left, count 5

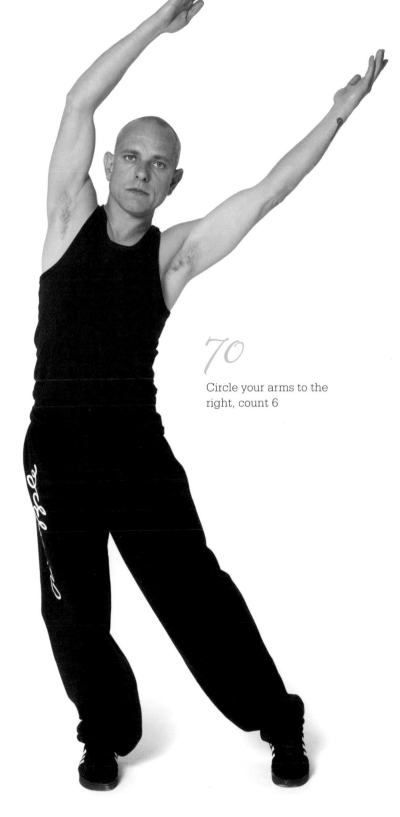

70

Circle your arms to the right, count 6

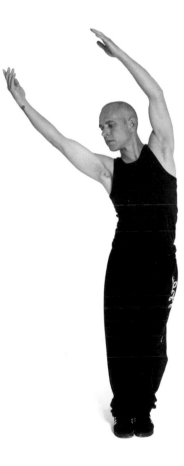

71

Bring your right foot to join your left and circle your arms to the left, also looking to the left, counts 7, hold 8.
Repeat steps 62 –71

acknowledgements

Arlene Phillips

Thanks to Giorgia Barberi, and Michael Ritchie for their endless support. To Alana Phillips for hair and make up. To Monsoon, Nike, Pineapple and Arlene Phillips for Marisota for the clothes. To Sue Fox for her way with words. Thanks, also, to Coco Crowley, without whose help and assistance this book would never have been made.

Publishers

The publishers would like to acknowledge the following copyright holders of the music to which the routines are set:

'Mamma Mia': Bocu Music Limited/Bocu (Abba Music)
'What a Feeling': Warner Chappell Morris Limited
'You Can't Stop the Beat': Songs of PEN UK
'We Will Rock You': Queen Music Limited
'We Go Together': Warner Chappell Morris Limited
'Fame': EMI United Partnership Limited
'Go Go Go Joseph': The Really Useful Group Limited
'Footloose': Sony/ATV Harmony UK/Universal/MCA Music Limited
'Night Fever': Universal Music Publishing International/Warner Chappell Morris Limited
'The Time of My Life': Sony/ATV Music Publishing UK/World Song Inc./Songs of PEN UK/EMI Music Publishing Limited